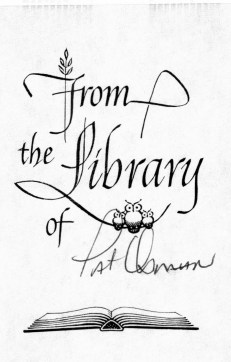

From
the Library
of
Pat Osmun

Planned Short-Term Treatment

Treatment Approaches in the Human Services

Francis J. Turner, Editor

Planned Short-Term Treatment

Richard A. Wells

THE FREE PRESS
A Division of Macmillan Publishing Co., Inc.
NEW YORK

Collier Macmillan Publishers
LONDON

The Free Press
A Division of Macmillan Publishing Co., Inc.
866 Third Avenue, New York, N. Y. 10022

Collier Macmillan Canada, Ltd.

Library of Congress Catalog Card Number: 81-67163

Printed in the United States of America

printing number

2 3 4 5 6 7 8 9 10

Library of Congress Cataloging in Publication Data

Wells, Richard A.
    Planned short-term treatment.

    (Treatment approaches in the human services)
    Includes bibliographical references and index.
    1. Psychotherapy, Brief. I. Title. II. Series.
[DNLM: 1. Psychotherapy, Brief. WM 420 W455p]
RC480.55.W44   616.89'14   81-67163
ISBN 0-02-934650-9   AACR2

To My Parents

Contents

Foreword

"Treatment Approaches in the Human Services" is the first series of professional texts to be prepared under the general auspices of social work. It is understandable that the editor and authors of this endeavor should be enthusiastic about its quality and prospects. But it is equally understandable that our enthusiasm is tempered with caution and prudence. There is a presumptuousness in attempting to be on the leading edge of thinking and aspiring to break new ground, and our professional experience urges us to be restrained.

The first suggestion for this series came from the editorial staff of The Free Press in the spring of 1975. At that time, the early responses to *Social Work Treatment** were available. It was clear from the responses that, useful as that book appeared to be, there was a wish and a need for more detail on each of the various thought systems covered, especially as regards their direct practice implications. These comments led to a proposal ffrom The Free Press that a series be developed that would expand the content of the individual chapters of *Social Work Treatment* into full-length books with the objective of providing a richer and fuller exposition of each system. This idea is still germane to the

---

*Francis J. Turner, ed., *Social Work Treatment* (New York: Free Press). The first edition was published in 1974 and the second in 1979.

series, but with the emergence of new thought systems and theories it has moved beyond the notion of expanding the chapters in the original collection. New thinking in the helping professions, the diversity of new demands, and the complexity of these demands have increased beyond the expectations of even the harbingers of the knowledge explosion of the early 1970s. No profession can or should stand still, and thus no professional literature can be static. It is our hope that this series will stay continuously current as it takes account of new ideas emerging from practice.

By design, this series has a strong orientation to social work. But it is not designed for social workers alone; it is also intended to be useful to our colleagues in other professions. The point has frequently been made that much of the conceptual base of social work practice has been borrowed and that social work has made few original contributions to other professions. That is no longer true. A principal assumption of this series is that social work must now accept the responsibility for making available to other professions its rich accumulation of theoretical concepts and therapeutic strategies.

The responsibility to share does not presume that professions with a healing and human-development commitment are moving to some commonality of identity and structure. In the next decade, we are probably going to see clearer rather than more obscure professional identities and more rather than less precise professional boundaries, derived not from different knowledge bases but from differential use of shared knowledge. If this prediction is valid, it follows that each profession must develop increased and enriched ways of making available to other professions its own expanding knowledge of the human condition.

Although the books in this series are written from the viewpoint of the clinician, they will be useful for the student-professional, the senior scholar, and the teacher of professionals as well. On the principle that no dynamic profession can tolerate division among its practitioners, theory builders, and teachers, each book is intended to be a bridging resource between practice and theory development. In directing this series to colleagues whose principal targets of practice are individuals, families, and groups, we take the other essential fields of practice as given. Thus the community-development, social-action, policy, research, and service-delivery roles of the helping professions are not specifically addressed in these books.

One of the risks of living and practicing in an environment characterized by pluralism in professions, practice styles, and theoretical orientations is that one may easily become doctrinaire in defending a particular perspective. Useful and important as is ongoing debate that leads to clarification of similarities and differences, overlaps and gaps in thought systems and theories, the authors of these books have been asked to minimize this function. That is, they are to analyze the conceptual base of their particular topic, identify its theoretical origins, and explain and describe its operationalization in practice, but avoid polemics in behalf of "their" system. Inevitably, some material of this type is needed for comparisons, but the aim is to make the books explicative rather than argumentative.

Although the series has a clear focus and explicit objectives, there is also a strong commitment that it be marked with a quality of development and evolution. It is hoped that we shall be responsive to changes in psychotherapeutic practice and to the needs of colleagues in practice and thus be ready to alter the format of subsequent books as may be necessary.

In a similar way, the ultimate number of books in the series has been left open. Viewing current practice in the late 1970s, it is possible to identify a large number of influential thought systems that need to be addressed. We can only presume that additional perspectives will emerge in the future. These will be addressed as the series continues, as will new developments or reformulations of existing practice perspectives.

The practice of psychotherapy and the wide spectrum of activities that it encompasses is a risky and uncertain endeavor. Clearly, we are just beginning a new era of human knowledge and improved clinical approaches and methods. At one time we were concerned because we knew so little; now we are concerned to use fully the rich progress that has been made in research, practice, and conceptualization. This series is dedicated to that task in the humble hope that it will contribute to man's concern for his fellows.

In addressing short-term treatment, Richard Wells' book makes an important contribution to the series. Short-term treatment, first viewed as a pragmatic yet second-best substitute for long-term treatment, has now taken its place as an approach to therapy (frequently the treatment of choice) for particular persons and situations. This is a dramatic and important shift from a perception among practitioners that if treatment was to be truly effective it needed to be long-term and in-depth. Interestingly, this belief in the inherent superiority of long-term treatment is still adhered to by some components of the helping professions.

This book gives further emphasis to the effectiveness of short-term treatment. Because the adherents of short-term treatment were aware that they were breaking away from tradition and orthodoxy in their writings, they have been careful to ensure that this method of treatment is subjected to careful scrutiny from a research perspective. Thus over the last ten years we have had continuing and solid evaluations of this approach that have strenthened the arguments in its support. Furthermore, this research stance has fortified the appreciation and importance of evaluative research for all approaches to treatment, not just short-term treatment.

In addition to the evaluative component, the short-term therapists have been thorough in identifying the components of treatment and the specific procedures that are employed in this approach. Richard Wells' book continues this tradition of thoroughness and gives us excellent details of individual practice techniques that make use of the cognitive affective and behavioral components of functioning.

In this book, Professor Wells strongly underscores the component of short-term treatment that stresses the need for a clear stipulation of the objectives, process, and techniques in each case. Besides giving the reader a rich presentation of this method, the author sets the material in the totality of the context of current practice emphasizing the responsibility of the therapist to be directive and precise and the need for the client to be actively involved in the problem-solving process by making full use of his or her resources and ability.

Although the book focuses on the single approach to practice of short-term treatment, the author stresses that it is an approach that draws on a plurality of thought system, thus once again stressing the advantages of interlocking treatment approaches to practice as well as the constant need to evaluate what it is we are doing. This will be a most useful book to practitioners and students alike from the perspective of thoroughness and clarity, with the additional benefit of a rich and broad-based bibliography.

FRANCIS J. TURNER

Preface and Acknowledgments

My intent in this work has been to present a model of planned short-term intervention that will be useful to the direct practitioner, in the front line of helping service, as well as to students and teachers of clinical practice. With the perspective of the clinician in mind I have emphasized the immediate details of practice and attempted to illustrate the manner in which technique and strategy must be adapted to the specific needs and unique characteristics of our clients. I hope that this view of practice will be useful to professional helpers of many disciplines and stimulate the growing interest in efficient and effective forms of clinical practice.

The theoretical underpinnings of the model will undoubtedly be seen as "eclectic" (although my own preference is for the term "pluralistic") but whatever the overall mix, the influence of concepts from social learning theory, crisis theory, and the interpersonal relationship framework will be clearly apparent. Actually theory, in the usual sense of abstract, general statements about the characteristics of troubled people or the principles of therapeutic treatment, has been one of my lesser concerns. I have attempted to draw upon the findings of the psychotherapy research literature, particularly as these bear upon the activities of the therapist and the outcomes of various interventions, and I believe that these findings should be regarded as the basic source of knowledge for practice. Any number of valuable clinical guidelines can be drawn from the research literature, provided that one is willing to make inferences beyond the raw data. Such extrapolation has been neglected by many clinical practitioners, who instead have tended to rely upon the testimony of authoritative figures in the field or their own immediate clinical experience.

It will be evident that I believe planned short-term treatment to be a clinical method of considerable scope and flexibility. It can be appropriately applied to a wide range of the problems in leving—personal, interpersonal, and social—that daily confront practitioners in family service agencies, mental health clinics, hospitals, and other such direct service settings. Obviously I have very definite convictions about the legitimacy and utility of time-limited intervention, but, in the spirit of Dr. Turner's remarks in the Foreword, I will mute any polemics and make my approach "explicative rather than argumentative."

Any author must acknowledge mutiple influences and, in the end, hope that these many debts are adequately documented in the citations and the reference list. Certain writers and researchers stand out, however, as enduring sources of knowledge and inspiration. Jerome Frank's seminol contributions to the psychotherapy literature have played a major role in shaping my thinking and practice. Social learning theory, particularly as explicated by Albert Bandura, has provided an integrative framework for my view of the principles of clinical assessment and intervention. Finally, William Reid's pioneering development of task-centered casework and his persistent labors in examining and validating many of the facets of short-term practice have been yet another significant influence.

A number of friends and colleagues also contributed. Jeanne Figurel and Larry Pacoe not only have enriched my appreciation of clinical practice, but both gave cogent critical readings to various drafts of the manuscript. At The Free Press, Gladys Topkis's skillful editing was invaluable, while Frank Turner's guidance, as general editor of the series, has been both encouraging and timely. Many others, including Patrick McNamee, Mary Page, Edward Zuckerman, Cheryl Pierce, and the late Lois Jaffe, through friendship and professional association, have added to this work and to my life. I am grateful for their help but must bear sole responsibility for the strengths or weaknesses of the final product.

In addition, the Maurice Falk Medical Foundation of Pittsburgh made funding available that greatly facilitated the final stages of preparation. Finally, my wife and children have shown a charitable forbearance toward an author's unfortunate tendency to become preoccupied with his writing task.

Richard A. Wells

Planned
Short-Term
Treatment

Chapter 1

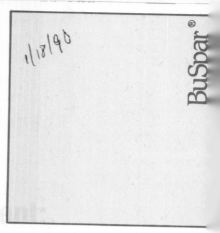

Short-Term Treatn

Overview and Evidence

If it were done when 'tis done, then 'twere well it were done quickly.

—William Shakespeare, *Macbeth*

The efficiency of therapeutic service has seldom been a burning issue in mental health circles. Whether one or another of the many helping approaches can deliver relief from suffering or restore function more promptly than others has not been a historic concern of the field. Perhaps Macbeth's injunction to himself, cited above, was ill-advised in his circumstances, yet a concern for speed does appear reasonable, at least in relation to helping troubled people. Effectiveness, of course, *has* been an issue. Does psychotherapy work? is the broad question. Despite sometimes strident voices to the contrary (Eysenck, 1952; Fischer, 1976), most clinicians have maintained that it does. However, combining these concerns for effectiveness and efficiency, one can easily arrive at the dilemma Garfield (1980) poses when he notes that the examination of therapeutic practice has largely concentrated on outcome effectiveness and ignored the question of time. He goes on to suggest that "from any vantage point . . . a brief but effective therapy would be much more utilitarian than

1

an equally effective therapy which requires a much longer period of time'' (p. 277).

These dual imperatives toward efficiency and effectiveness have undoubtedly played a role in motivating the increasing numbers of practitioners in the helping professions who are turning to short-term treatment methods as an accepted and in many instances a preferred mode of intervention. Such authors as Parad (1971) and Reid and Epstein (1972) in social work; Barten (1969), Langsley (1978), and Marmor (1979) in psychiatry; and Butcher and Koss (1978) in clinical psychology have all documented this burgeoning trend.

There is even reason to believe that in the daily realities of practice relatively brief rather than long-term treatment is actually becoming the norm. In a later section of this chapter I will examine several recent large-scale surveys of clinical practice that offer support for this viewpoint. Initially, however, it will be best to simply review the various factors that have promoted the present interest in brief intervention and present an overview of the principles of such clinical practice. Additional sections will examine certain theoretical and philosophical issues related to its use and discuss the particular clientele most suited to brief therapeutic approaches. A final section will review the substantial body of research evidence supporting the effectiveness of short-term intervention.

> *Short-term treatment,* as I shall use this term, *refers to a group (or family) of related therapeutic interventions in which the helper deliberately and planfully limits both the goals and the duration of contact.*

The goals of therapy are almost always explicitly contracted with the client and directly related to the specific life difficulties the client desires to solve. The length of intervention is determined by the clinical judgment of the therapist but is usually between three and fifteen sessions. Within these parameters of purpose and time many variations are possible, and certain of these will be discussed in later chapters. At this point, however, this definition will serve as a rough guideline to the most distinctive characteristics of short-term methodology.

The Impetus Toward Short-Term Intervention

The development of community mental health facilities, particularly during the late 1960s, placed enormous pressure on the helping professions to meet expanding demands for service. This pressure has continued—even as governmental funding diminishes—and clinics and agencies must still strive to meet expanded client loads despite depleted staffs. Thus interest has become directed toward finding interventive methods requiring less staff time yet still offering satisfactory levels of outcome.

As a further consequence of the movement into community mental health, another factor has become more and more apparent: not only do the existing methods not meet the need for effectiveness and efficiency, but in many instances the clients do not want the methods. Thus as service has been increasingly offered to lower socioeconomic and working-class groups, it has been found that their concern is with the reduction of current social and interpersonal stress—with ridding themselves of distressing or incapacitating difficulties in daily living. Such problems may, at times, appear mundane but can represent very real dilemmas for the prospective client.

Alice Martin, a nineteen-year-old single woman, was referred by the nurse practitioner who was caring for her during her second pregnancy. The nurse expressed concern that Miss Martin, who was six months pregnant, was having difficulty in managing her day-by-day activities, as her boyfriend, on whom she had depended a good deal, had recently been sent to prison. An initial interview with Miss Martin revealed that she saw herself experiencing problems in two areas: first, she was receiving welfare payments and was finding it difficult to budget her money; and second, she was worried about child care and transportation arrangements at the time of labor and delivery but was reluctant to approach her family for help.

A difficulty for the practitioner has been that methods specific to such immediate goals have been lacking. The conventional clinical philosophy has been to disparage such problems as mere "symptoms." While middle-class clients have often been willing to accept this view, lower socioeconomic clients have been notoriously reluctant.

There has also been a clearer recognition that traditional treatment approaches do not meet the emerging need for efficient yet effective methods. Conventional clinical lore, for example, has cherished the notion of highly trained professionals involved in long periods of treatment with clients who are verbal, voluntary, introspective, and, in general, well motivated. As Marmor (1979) points out, the "vast majority of American psychiatrists are still heavily committed to a one-to-one model of dynamic psychotherapy" (p. 149), an approach which places particular stress on these desirable client characteristics and typically envisages a lengthy period of therapeutic contact. Such approaches are obviously unrealistic and unworkable in settings where the modal client is much more likely to be a rather unsophisticated individual with perhaps high school education and from a working-class background. Unless one is prepared to screen out droves of clients as unsuitable, it is imperative that other interventive methods be found.

Marmor (1979) goes on to suggest that "we are living in the midst of a major psychotherapeutic revolution" (p. 149) marked by the emergence of numerous new therapies of varying degrees of merit. His discussion of short-term dynamic psychotherapy not only describes the intellectual ferment that has been a catalyst in the development of brief treatment but, perhaps even more compellingly, identifies some cogent economic factors related to its growth. He predicts:

> At the same time the development of third-party payers, together with the imminence of some form of national health insurance, places psychiatrists under pressure to find shorter, more broadly applicable, and more efficient techniques of therapy or risk exclusion from these programs for fiscal reasons. As a consequence, we

can anticipate that the briefer techniques of group therapy, behavioral therapy, and family therapy will emerge more strongly in the years ahead [p. 149].

Gerald Zuk (1978), in a recent discussion of trends in family therapy, has emphasized a similar theme. He points out that one of the significant changes in the practice of family therapy in the past few years has been a movement toward short-term contact. He contends that the majority of families are prepared to allow therapeutic access for only a limited period of time and that the therapist must capitalize on this apparent restriction by utilizing an appropriate methodology.

Zuk places considerable emphasis on the importance of engagement into therapy, especially where motivation is weak or ambivalent. I will place a similar stress on the engagement aspects of planned short-term treatment, which are examined in some detail in Chapters 4 and 5, on the initial interview. As well as exploring the issue of inadequate motivation, these chapters will highlight the need for a focused and systematic approach to initiating brief therapy.

There is a good deal of empirical evidence, however, that whatever the modality of intervention, many clients do not stay in treatment if emphasis is placed on such broad concepts as personality reorganization or overall personal growth in the context of long-term contact. Where systematic studies have been conducted, it has been found that mental health clinics and family service agencies have appallingly high drop-out rates. As many as 80 percent of cases are seen for less than six interviews. Garfield (1971, 1980), for example, has reviewed the studies substantiating this finding across all psychotherapeutic settings, while Beck and Jones (1973), Howard and Libbie Parad (1968), and Verny (1970) offer data on family service, child guidance, and mental health clinics, respectively.

The large percentage of cases involving fewer than six interviews suggests that a great deal of *unplanned* short-term treatment takes place. On the one hand, contact between helper and client may be brief because the process founders. However good the intentions of the therapist, nothing really helpful transpires and the client withdraws from the relationship. On the other hand, it may well be that the client has benefited from even this short encounter and has therefore chosen, unilaterally, to terminate active treatment. In either case, there is no doubt that most therapeutic contact is relatively brief, and it behooves us to examine the meaning of this phenomenon.

Furthermore, research on crisis (Caplan, 1964; Hansell, 1975) has strongly suggested that many people come for help at a point when they are in severe distress. As a crisis tends to resolve itself, for better or worse, within a relatively short period of time, it is apparent that helping services must be devised that work effectively within this natural time limit. Access to many clients is comparatively brief, and the therapist must be prepared to work in the most helpful manner possible within these limitations rather than futilely wish that there was more time.

Finally, where short-term and long-term approaches have been empirically compared, there has been a consistent finding with significant client populations that they are equal in results. (A later section of this chapter will review this research.) Short-term treatment, in other words, is not necessarily a second-rate substitute for long-term treatment but in many instances is capable of delivering as much service in less time. This, of course, has many implications for practitioners, agencies, funding sources, and, most importantly, clients and their right to both effective and efficient service.

An Overview of Short-Term Treatment

The theoretical base of the model of planned short-term treatment presented in this book represents an integration of two major influences in the helping field, namely, the behavior modification methods deriving from social learning theory, and the time-limited approaches stemming from the study of crisis. Behavior therapy has shown that people can achieve meaningful changes in their lives through structured methods that emphasize the identification of desired behaviors, the step-by-step acquisition of change through imitation and practice, and the generalizing of such change into real life via homework tasks and assignments. Crisis theory and intervention not only have identified the stressful life events that frequently motivate people to seek help but have highlighted the significance of time in the process of change. That is to say, a crisis can be seen as a time-limited event in the life of its victim which will resolve itself (for better or worse) unless effective help is received within its natural life span.

Two further conceptual frameworks implicitly influence the model of short-term intervention to be presented. Ego psychology, with its emphasis on the characteristics of human functioning in its conscious and socially adaptive manifestations, is, of course, a pervasive influence in the helping field. Similarly, interpersonal relationship theory (plus its almost unacknowledged transformation into much current family therapy theory and practice) is yet another powerful force with many of its viewpoints so permeating practice that they are taken for granted. Selected aspects of these four frameworks of clinical thought will be considered in greater detail in Chapter 2. In this overview I will concentrate upon the first two, which have most obviously (and recently) influenced brief therapy.

Both behavioral modification and crisis intervention are aimed at instigating change in the current life of the individual seeking help. They share the common assumption that human difficulties are most usefully conceptualized as problems in living—disruptions in the person's daily life, dissatisfaction with the quality or quantity of interpersonal relationship, deficits in the essential social skills needed to manage one's life—and that the focus of treatment should be on remedying these gaps. Short-term treatment is a deliberate and concentrated method of meeting such goals and is intended to be both a practical and an accessible means of helping large groups of people who otherwise would have little suitable therapeutic service at their command.

It should be noted, however, that although it is influenced by certain facets of crisis theory, short-term therapy is not identical with crisis intervention. The various short-term approaches can be seen as a related family of interventions, incorporating crisis intervention as an important subtype but including techniques, strategies, and goals that move beyond the crisis formulation. These include interventions aimed at promoting change in specific areas of personal and interpersonal functioning, methods of imparting important social knowledge and skills, and, in other instances, approaches designed to assist an individual in solving a particularly difficult life problem.

Crisis intervention typically aims at restoring the precrisis equilibrium of the sufferer. Brief treatment, in contrast, often attempts to develop new learnings and skills that will enable the individual to progress beyond his or her original status. Crisis work is primarily supportive and ameliorative—and highly valuable within these designated parameters. Short-term treatment, in the broader dimensions that will be presented in this work, is designed to engage the client in problem-resolution or change efforts with wider-ranging implications. A further important distinction is that crisis intervention emphasizes the individual or family in acute emotional distress, whereas short-term treatment is suitable for a range of clients whose affective state may be much less profoundly disturbed.

In practice, short-term intervention involves the employment of specific personal and behavioral change methods, over an explicitly defined period of time, with the objective of bringing about positive changes in the client's current life. In addition, the helping process is intended to relieve the often painful stress and demoralization that accompany disruptions and difficulties in the client's intimate interpersonal relationships, important social roles, and significant personal functioning. Drop-outs and unplanned terminations decrease markedly with this dual emphasis on time and reality.

The therapist and client jointly select one or two major areas of difficulty as the target of the helping intervention and agree to work on these problems for a planned period of time. It is usually the responsibility of the therapist to choose the particular change techniques that are judged to be most pertinent to achieving the desired goal and to guide and encourage the client in their application. The change methods employed are structured, in the sense of comprising a series of steps (or phases) that break the process of change into component parts and guide the activities of both helper and client. Many such techniques are now available in the clinical literature, covering a wide range of common social and interpersonal situations. The therapist's activities throughout the helping process are directed toward (1) making problem and goal definitions as clear as possible, (2) supporting the client in systematic, step-by-step problem solving, and (3) using the pressures of an explicit time limit as a key factor toward change.

Looking upon time as a critical element in the process of short-term intervention, it is possible to conceptualize the contact between helper and client as comprising three distinct phases, each with distinct temporal boundaries:

1. The first phase consists of one or two interviews in which problems and goals are defined and an explicit contract is negotiated.
2. This is followed by the main period of intervention (up to fifteen sessions), in which selected change strategies are utilized and which concludes with an evaluative termination interview.
3. The third phase involves a follow-up interview, two to four months later. This interview, initiated by the therapist, is utilized to review the client's current status.

The therapist not only spells out the time dimensions of each of these phases to the client but adjusts the therapeutic effort to fit within the defined boundaries. This results in highly positive pressures on both therapist and client to identify the most pressing problem(s) and to work productively to bring about the desired changes. Implicit in the short-term helping process is the belief that change is most likely to ensue from a concentrated focus on a single but significant problem in living (and, conversely, the belief that much natural problem solving is weakened by attempting to deal with too many difficulties simultaneously). In order to emphasize this process, the helper will insist that the client with multiple problems choose the one or two of highest priority for intervention.

Most short-term work terminates at the end of the contracted period (plus the designated follow-up), but it should be noted that it is always possible for therapist and client to negotiate, at the end of a particular helping sequence, an agreement to concentrate on a new problem area. Additionally, if short-term treatment does not achieve its goals within the expected time, therapist and client may agree to move into a further time-limited contract or, in some cases, extended treatment.

A Prospective Clientele

Many helping methods have unfortunately based their techniques and strategies on clinical experience and research with a socially and emotionally advantaged clientele. Indeed, by their very nature a number of therapies either directly or indirectly screen out prospective clients who are not intelligent, highly motivated, relatively affluent, and managing their current lives well enough that they are willing to enter a lengthy therapeutic experience with little immediate hope of benefit.

Yet there is no doubt that a great many very ordinary people seek help only at a point where emotional stress has assumed major proportions. Such potential clients have little concept of therapy as a process aimed at wide-ranging personality change over a period of years and tend to drop out of treatment rather

rapidly when its goals appear vague or irrelevant and the expected time commitment seems endless. Other clients become dependent upon the helping process and stay within its protective confines long past any point of real gain.

There are large numbers of people to whom the services of private practitioners—whatever their discipline—are simply not accessible. Partly this is a question of money: many struggling middle-class, lower-middle-class, or blue-collar clients (to say nothing of the poor) cannot afford the fee of the private practitioner. Furthermore, the expectations that these clients bring into the therapeutic situation are frequently far different from those of the conventional therapist. They do not want to change their total personality; rather, they want to learn how to consistently discipline and nurture a difficult child. They do not want to expand their intellectual and emotional awareness, but instead are concerned with how to reduce the quarreling and dissatisfaction of a painful marriage. These are legitimate requests—not "symptoms" of something else—and need to be met with respect, concern and effective helping from the clinical practitioner.

Mrs. Antonini phoned a family service agency to request help for her husband, whom she described as extremely upset and anxious about difficulties he was encountering at work. She accompanied him to the initial interview and they were seen together.

A neatly dressed, rather conventional working-class couple in their middle twenties, both were ill at ease as the session began. Finally, with obvious discomfort and embarrassment, Mr. Antonini described how his co-workers at the factory where he was employed had been verbally harassing him for the past year or two. The harassment consisted mainly of remarks and innuendos to the effect that he was effeminate or even homosexual. These stemmed, Mr. Antonini believed, from an incident where he had been overheard masturbating in the company washroom. Mr. Antonini had been able to make only the most ineffectual responses to these sallies; his major coping device was to avoid contact with the chief instigators of the ridicule. He had become increasingly upset about the situation, but only recently had he been able to confide these difficulties to his wife. He felt some relief from having shared his feelings but at the same time expressed an almost desperate concern to find some way of managing the continuing harassment.

I will return to this case in greater detail in a later chapter. At this point it will be sufficient to note that although a complex of psychological, emotional, and social factors are evident in the difficult situation facing Mr. Antonini, the focus of brief treatment was on responding to his urgent request for some tangible ways of coping with a situation that was both deeply troubling to him and threatening his ability to continue to earn a living.

From this stance the helping practitioner is not a healer, diagnosing and treating "mental illness," moving from symptoms to underlying disease or pathology in some conjectured analogy to the model of medical practice. Rather, the helper becomes in many instances an *educator* (Guerney et al., 1971) teaching needed skills in living or, in other instances, an *expert problem solver* (Haley, 1976) guiding clients in their efforts to cope with the intricacies and frustrations of the human condition.

Although I will frequently use the term "client" (and very occasionally "patient") in referring to persons in need of skilled helping, one can gain a very different and highly useful perspective by thinking of such people as *customers* or *consumers* of helping services (Lazare et al., 1972, 1975a, 1975b). From this vantage point the request of the customer becomes critical and must be clearly understood if a suitable helping service is to be delivered. Lazare and his colleagues contend that the professional often mishears the troubled person's request or casts it in an entirely inappropriate mold because of an overemphasis on the traditional norms of clinical practice.

Rabkin (1977) makes a similar point when he notes how most initial interviews have been designed to determine the suitability of the person, as potential patient, for treatment. He argues that identifying the request of the client, and then devising an intervention suitable to meeting this request, is the essence of brief therapy. This approach, and the insights offered by Lazare's emphasis on the client as customer, will be developed in greater depth in later chapters on the process and goals of the initial interview.

The Confusions of Practice: Proliferation and Neglect

Adding to the difficulty and uncertainty for the practitioner—whether beginning or experienced—in conceptualizing the client's troubles as problems in living has been a prolonged, contentious, and ultimately irreconcilable dispute within the helping professions about the proper method and goal of therapeutic intervention. The dispute has not been as much between the three major helping professions of social work, psychology, and psychiatry (although there are certainly some differences in the objectives of these disciplines) as it has been among the numerous schools and modes of therapy, each offering apparently different theories of change, varying techniques for inducing change, and in many instances unique modes of service delivery. Even the most casual student of psychotherapy requires little convincing on the essential point—methods of therapy have proliferated to an almost bewildering degree, and along with this proliferation the goals of helping have become exceedingly obscured.

Within this context of dispute and disagreement it might seem hopelessly naive and futile to offer yet another version of helping methods. Such an attempt could appear even more fruitless when certain of its major premises—an emphasis on problems in living, specific goals, structured procedures, and time-limited contact—run so counter to many of the prevalent beliefs in the helping professions. Despite this sense of swimming upstream, at least in regard to apparent norms and practices, there is sufficient reason to believe that much helping is ineffectual, that large groups of needy people are being neglected, and that there is considerable virtue (both empirically and practically) in concreteness, simplicity, and brevity; and the effort, therefore, must be made.

Philosophically, much of the rationale for a structured, goal-oriented, short-term approach to helping practice lies in the consonance of such an approach with the common motivations that characterize many consumers of such services. People approach a helping source for a wide variety of reasons, with extremely varying degrees of willingness and unwillingness and with many different expectations. Certainly variability is the rule rather than the exception. Yet there are commonalities marking the entry into the client role, and the essential skill of the helper at this fundamental level lies in recognizing and, in negotiation with the seeker of help, articulating this common core. Possibly the most important commonality lies in the concern (in many cases even anguish and despair) of the client about the problems he or she is experiencing in the conduct of daily life. This may be seen in the disruptions of feeling that affect, for example, job performance or even such natural functions as sleeping or eating. In other instances the intimate relationships in which the potential client is engaged may be dissatisfying or conflicted. For others the resources needed to make life more fulfilling—for some to simply make it bearable—may be seemingly unavailable. These are but examples of the life difficulties and dilemmas that impel people to seek help. From the point of view of the consumer of service the helping intervention must provide solutions to such common problems, and this, of course, is the explicit focus of the short-term approaches.

The short-term practitioner attempts to understand the client's request, to make it more specific, if need be, and to design an intervention that will promote the changes desired by the client. Such a direct approach to helping places considerable pressure on the helper to be highly knowledgeable about interventive techniques that will bring about specific changes or teach essential skills. Short-term treatment also places pressure on both client and helper to work systematically and purposefully toward these chosen goals.

All of this emphasizes a much more active and directive role for the helper than the conventional approaches have usually taught or condoned. In addition, there is considerable stress in brief therapy on the evaluation of treatment, not only throughout the process of intervention but also at termination and follow-up points after active contact has been completed. Only through forthright and responsible self-examination by the helper can the rights of the client—the consumer of helping services—be safeguarded and the helper's own professional growth promoted.

Short-Term Treatment and the Realities of Clinical Practice

A later section of this chapter will present a range of data supporting the position that short-term treatment is therapeutically effective. Its cost and time efficiency are obvious. Earlier sections have attempted to point out that there are also cogent social and moral reasons for its employment. Yet the prevailing belief has been that most clinicians prefer (and actually practice) long-term treatment. Several recent studies of clinical practice, across all the major helping professions, contradict this belief and even suggest that time-limited intervention may be becoming the accepted norm of practice. A major study by Beck and Jones, published in 1973, offers such a picture of clinical practice in social work, while Langsley, in 1978, and Koss, in 1979, offer similar reports on the clinical work of psychiatrists and psychologists, respectively.

The study of social work practice conducted by Beck and Jones (1973) was based on an examination of 3,596 cases from a nationwide sample of family service agencies, gathered in 1970. The authors compared these findings with a similar study conducted in 1960 and found that for interventions with relationship and personality problems (77 percent of the agencies' caseload) there was a marked trend toward increased utilization of short-term treatment, particularly for child-related problems. Perhaps the most startling finding is contained in an obscure footnote (1973, p. 188, note 30) which states that the short-term cases in their sample averaged *five* sessions while the continued service cases averaged *nine* interviews! That a nationwide sample of "continued service" cases falls squarely within what are usually considered short-term time limits certainly reinforces the notion that a good deal of brief treatment is being given in an unacknowledged manner.

In a more recent article, Langsley (1978) describes the results of a survey of psychiatric practice conducted over a six-month period in 1974. In this study both private and clinic psychiatrists reported on the diagnosis and treatment of all cases where intervention was considered complete and terminated with the practitioner's agreement. A total of 4,072 cases were reported by 147 private practitioners and 51 clinic psychiatrists. It is important to note that these were all cases in which treatment had been concluded; the study did not include consultations, incomplete treatment, or unplanned drop-outs.*

It was found that the median number of office visits, across all diagnoses, was 12.8 for private psychiatrists and 10.3 for the clinic practitioners. Thus, in terms of length of treatment, there was little difference between private and institutional practice; therapists in both settings were apparently conducting a sizable amount of relatively brief treatment. As Langsley points out, contrary to popular belief, psychiatrists as a group do not predominantly practice long-term treatment; private psychiatrists, in particular, frequently utilize brief interventions; and even the more severe disorders do not necessarily receive lengthy treatment. (If anything, the trend was for such milder diagnostic categories as "situational disturbance of childhood and adolescence" to receive longer contact.)

Finally, Koss (1979) examined the characteristics of all the

---

*It should also be noted that Langsley's major purpose in conducting the survey was not to document the prevalence of short-term treatment, but to ease the worries of third-party payers who have thought that private psychiatric treatment was predominantly long term. As the earlier quotation from Marmor indicated, a recurring fear among psychiatrists is the apprehension that they may be excluded from the rich lode of a national health insurance.

cases seen over a year's time at a private clinic staffed by seven psychologists. The 100 subjects included in the study comprised all persons who requested and attended at least one psychotherapeutic session during this time period. The central finding was that length of treatment for 79 percent of the sample was twenty interviews or less. Koss points out that this service utilization pattern is little different from that of clients in public agencies and underscores the need to "continue to develop and evaluate treatment approaches designed to utilize effectively the brief time clients, even the most socially advantaged, will remain in psychotherapy" (p. 211).

It appears unnecessary, then, to try to persuade practitioners to do more short-term treatment when, in fact, the bulk of actual practice is already relatively brief. The real difficulty may lie in the cognitive dissonance this creates for the therapist who, on the one hand, has been taught to believe in the superiority of extended treatment and yet must grapple with the reality of a practice that is largely brief contact. The purpose of examining the principles and techniques of short-term intervention in this work is not to change practice in any major way; this has apparently taken place. The need, rather, is to explicate the empirical, theoretical, and technological foundations of time-limited intervention so as to improve the quality of such practice and reinforce its *explicit* acceptability among practitioners.

Empirical Support for Short-Term Approaches

Reid (1978) has argued that one of the essential values in a client-oriented approach to clinical practice is "the supremacy of research-based knowledge over knowledge acquired from other sources, such as practice wisdom or untested theory" (p. 5). I will take a similar stance in advocating that the practice of therapeutic helping must first turn to general principles, derived from the large body of research data concerning the process and outcome of therapeutic intervention, before even considering the many theories available. Thus, rather than examine theory first and then attempt to find data to support it, I will reverse this process and employ the findings of research as a source of generalization about effective practice. The several theoretical frameworks that I will review in Chapter 2 will be regarded as supplementary to the empirical findings and useful mainly in articulating and guiding the artful application of these research-based findings into the immediate practice context.

During the past decade a series of critical reviews have appeared which have attempted to compress the findings of psychotherapy research into a more manageable form. For example, analyses have been published which examine the process and outcome of therapeutic intervention in such specific problem areas as school phobias (Doleys, 1977) or marital conflict (Beck, 1975) with particular modalities of treatment such as family therapy (Wells and Dezen, 1978) and group therapy (Bednar and Lawlis, 1971) or with such identifiable client populations as the low socioeconomic (Lorion, 1978) or chronic alcoholics (Baekland et al., 1975). Besides these specific surveys, a number of writers have surveyed the overall findings of psychotherapy research in an effort to make these more accessible to the practitioner.*

A broad consideration of the data from both the general and specific reviews supports the position that short-term interventions are generally as effective as lengthier interventions with similar client populations. Where direct comparisons have been made between time-limited and extended treatment approaches, the consistent finding has been that the recipients of brief intervention make as much gain as those receiving lengthier treatment (Frank, 1979; Garfield, 1980; Luborsky et al., 1975; Strupp, 1978). This finding does not mean that extended treatment should

---

*Discussion in this section will draw upon such major reviews as Bergin (1971), Bergin and Lambert (1978), Frank (1979), Garfield (1980), Kazdin and Wilson (1978), Luborsky et al. (1971, 1975), Meltzoff and Kornreich (1970), Parloff (1979), and Strupp (1978).

not be practiced, but emphasizes that there is a need to identify those individuals or problems requiring this type of help, as the majority of clients benefit as much from a limited intervention.

There are a number of areas in which the evidence for the effectiveness of brief treatment is especially strong. These include conflicted marital relationships, the emotional and social problems of children and adolescents, crises of individuals and families, and, broadly speaking, many other aspects of disturbed social and interpersonal relationships. Quite aside from these specific areas, it may be surprising to find that short-term treatment has been attempted—although, admittedly, with varying degrees of success—with almost every type of client and problem known to the mental health professions (Wells, 1976).

For example, recent reviews of marital therapy by Dorothy Beck (1975) and Alan Gurman (1975) have both emphasized the efficacy of short-term interventions in treating marital conflict. Gurman notes that the cases in the studies he reviewed averaged a little more than sixteen interviews yet achieved an improvement rate of 76 percent. He points out:

> We have absolutely no research evidence on the effects of long-term couples therapy. This does not necessarily imply that some couples may not require extended therapy but, rather, that the burden of proof of what additional gains may be found in therapy of long duration rests with those clinicians who would advocate such practice [p. 421].

Similar reviews of short-term treatment with individuals have been conducted by Barten (1969), Reid and Shyne (1969), Reid and Epstein (1972), and, most recently, Butcher and Koss (1978). These reviews document the numerous studies which support the effectiveness of brief intervention with a wide range of social and interpersonal problems in adult and child clients.

Moreover, there is also highly suggestive evidence from studies of the therapeutic process that the most significant changes occur early in treatment and are followed by a period of diminishing effectiveness. Indeed, Meltzoff and Kornreich (1970), in their massive review of the outcome of therapeutic intervention of all types, remark that "psychotherapy, when successful, achieves its major gains relatively early" (p. 357). This further buttresses the short-term theme of vigorous, brief intervention.

I will not attempt to survey the total body of research studies that have examined the results of short-term treatment. The reviews noted above do this job quite adequately, and Reid (1978) succinctly summarizes the major findings. Several major studies will be described, however, in order to provide the reader with some picture of the supporting evidence available and, in particular, to highlight the studies that have dealt specifically with problems and client populations of relevance to clinical practice in mental health, family service, and child guidance settings.

In one of the landmark studies of time-limited approaches, Howard and Libbie Parad (1968) examined the results of 1,656 cases seen in planned short-term treatment in a nationwide sample drawn from family service agencies and child guidance clinics. The problems dealt with ranged over a wide spectrum of marital, family, parent-child, personal, and behavioral problems common to such agencies. The Parads note that 86 percent of the cases were handled within the planned time limits. This supports the view that in such settings only a minority of clients (14 percent in this large-scale survey) will require lengthier treatment. This finding, in other words, strongly suggests that large numbers of the problem situations typical of such settings can be managed within a short-term framework.

From evaluations completed by both therapists and clients it was found that the target problem improved in 65 to 75 percent of the cases (with the clients giving the higher rating). Similarly, better coping with stress was reported in 65 percent of the therapist ratings and 75 percent of the client evaluations. These assessments are certainly indicative of a very potent method at work and demonstrate its effectiveness across a broad range of human problems.

In the Beck and Jones (1973) large-scale nationwide study noted earlier, the outcome of over 3,000 family service cases was evaluated by both counselors and clients. These comprised the mixture of parent-child, marital, and personal problems typical of such settings. In all of the comparisons between planned short-term treatment and continued service, the brief intervention attained equal results or was slightly superior. Even if the outcomes are considered only equivalent, Beck and Jones point out that this was achieved in considerably less time than with the extended service. They also found that clients were significantly less likely to drop out of the short-term treatment prematurely.

In another important study Reid and Shyne (1969) randomly assigned 120 family service agency cases, experiencing predominantly marital and parent-child difficulties, to either short-term treatment (limited to eight sessions) or an open-ended approach. Such measures as client and therapist evaluations, research interview questionnaires, and ratings by independent judges were used to assess results at both termination and a follow-up point. Like other comparative studies of short-term and extended treatment, this study found the brief intervention to be at least as effective as the longer approach, and in some categories more effective.

Examining the effects of short-term methods with over 1,000 cases in a child guidance clinic, Leventhal and Weinberger (1975) found that short-term treatment produced improvement rates equal to (or better than) the long-term treatment approaches the clinic had previously employed. As in the Beck and Jones study noted earlier, this large-scale study also reported that drop-out rates were greatly reduced.

Finally, Sloane and his colleagues (1975) compared the outcome of both behavioral and psychodynamic short-term approaches (each employing a three-month time limit) with the changes occurring in an untreated control group. Their patients were moderately to severely disturbed adults seen as outpatients in a community mental health center. Results were evaluated using therapist, patient, and significant other (spouse, family member, etc.) ratings of change. In addition, a comprehensive evaluation interview was conducted by an independent clinician.

All of these assessments were carried out before and after treatment and at one- and two-year follow-up points. Highly experienced, skilled therapists were employed in both treatment conditions.

This study is widely regarded as probably the best-designed examination of therapeutic practice that has been carried out, and its findings have implications for both short-term therapy and clinical intervention generally. Significant and substantial levels of improvement were found in both the treated groups at termination in comparison with the nontreated clients, indicating that therapeutic intervention (at least in the short run) does induce meaningful change. The behavioral and psychodynamic approaches were equally effective, although, contrary to popular opinion, the behavioral approach was effective across a wider range of client disturbance. The psychodynamic intervention was most effective with mildly disturbed individuals, whereas the behavioral methods helped those with both mild and severe dysfunction. These results must be tempered, however, by the finding that by the one- and two-year follow-up points all patients, whether treated or untreated, were substantially improved. This supports the general viewpoint (Bergin and Lambert, 1978; Frank, 1979; Parloff, 1979) that any psychotherapeutic intervention operates most effectively in the early phases of intervention and that, beyond this point, natural remedial factors will promote positive change whether or not the individual is treated.

Clinicians have been concerned about the durability of the effects of time-limited intervention. Are gains from brief therapy ephemeral and liable to dissipate rapidly once therapeutic contact ends? A number of studies of short-term treatment (for example, Langsley et al., 1971; Keilson et al., 1979; Reid and Shyne, 1969; Sloane et al., 1975; Wells et al., 1977) have included follow-up evaluations in their research design. Thus client status has been assessed anywhere from four months to two and one-half years after the conclusion of treatment. The consistent finding has been that the gains derived from short-term treatment may show some slight decline at follow-up, but this is no different from the findings shown by any other therapeutic approach. Once again, the empirical data emphasize *equality* with other approaches.

Thus it is apparent that short-term treatment has been widely tested with large numbers of cases in a variety of therapeutic settings. The approach can be as readily utilized with the problems of children and their parents as it can with the difficulties of individual adults. It can be adapted to the interpersonal complexities of family and marital conflict as well as to the more individually focused problems of people in severe personal distress. Careful evaluations of effectiveness, using all of the methods currently available, support the position that brief intervention can deliver results at least equal to much longer interventions.

All of this establishes, moreover, that short-term treatment is not a passing fad, but a serious and purposeful therapeutic endeavor. This is not to say that brief intervention should always be employed. There are undoubtedly clients who, as the Parad and Parad (1968) study reported, need a longer intervention. However, on the basis of the accumulated evidence available, I believe that the following position is empirically justified:

> *Short-term treatment should be considered the treatment of choice in such settings as mental health clinics and child guidance and family service agencies except where there is specific empirical evidence that a particular client group or presenting problem requires lengthier treatment.*

This, of course, does not preclude the possibility that certain individuals, couples, or families will need more extended treatment, but it suggests that the way to find this out is after a trial of brief intervention has not achieved the desired results. The research evidence supports the position that, in a large proportion of instances, brief intervention will bring about as much change as a longer intervention. Moreover, the *equality* of outcome that has been demonstrated is being achieved in less time, and with less cost, not only for the client but in relation to scarce personnel resources.

Plan of the Book

The succeeding chapters of this book will attempt three main tasks: (1) to outline a theoretical foundation for short-term treatment, (2) to examine the process and goals of the initial phase of brief intervention, and (3) to explore certain of the major strategies of change employed by the short-term therapist.

Thus, Chapters 2 and 3 can be seen as interrelated. In the first of these chapters I will examine several theoretical frameworks that have proved useful in conceptualizing the process of short-term treatment and guiding its application. This chapter will present an eclectic approach to theory on the ground that there is no compelling reason to choose one theoretical orientation over another—all have their advantages and disadvantages for the practitioner. On the other hand, Chapter 3 will take a more pragmatic viewpoint and describe several short-term cases in detail, in order to give the reader a clearer picture of the characteristics and typical course of this form of therapeutic helping.

Chapters 4 and 5 will then examine the initial interview in depth. The theme of engagement into treatment will be emphasized, and the active and direct role of the practitioner within this process will be highlighted. Because of the brief therapist's deliberate restriction of time and selection of a limited focus, the skillful management of the first contact is critical to effective short-term therapy.

Finally, Chapters 6, 7, 8, and 9 are concerned with the implementation of change. The clinical application of behavior enactment (or rehearsal) methods and various types of task assignment will be examined and illustrated. These change strategies are particularly useful in short-term treatment because of their active nature and immediate application to problems in living. Chapters in this section will also discuss social skill training approaches and the recently developed cognitive restructuring methods. Skill training, derived from behaviorally oriented sources, emphasizes the step-by-step acquisition of facility in such socially important areas as communication, affiliation, assertion, and intimate relationships. Cognitive restructuring, a more recent development, draws upon a wide range of theoretical influences and emphasizes techniques for altering negative self-evaluations, excessively high performance standards, irrational beliefs, and the like.

The concluding chapter surveys a number of philosophical, theoretical, and practical issues in the utilization of short-term treatment in clinical practice. It should be noted, finally, that throughout this book brief therapy will be considered mainly in relation to one-to-one intervention. Although time-limited treatment has frequently been used in marital, family, and group modes, my preference in this work is to concentrate upon a single client, in keeping with the short-term philosophy of deliberately focusing upon a major area of concern in order to do a thorough job in this selected area.

Chapter 2

Pluralism in Practice: Theoretical Influences

> Everybody *has won, and all must have prizes.*
> —*Alice's Adventures in Wonderland*

Clinical practitioners in the helping professions are concerned with three essential questions about human behavior. First, how do problems in living develop? Why does one individual become embroiled in difficulties while another individual, often apparently similar in most respects, copes quite successfully? Second, once a problem in living has developed, what maintains its existence? Given that such difficulties are by their very nature emotionally stressful and frequently impede individuals in the realization of important goals, what tends to support their continuance? Third, how does an individual change from a problematic to a nonproblematic status? Even more specifically, what part can the helping professional play in stimulating such processes of change?

The most important practical question for the clinician is how to bring about tangible and beneficial change in the client's life. In contrast to the pure scientist or the academician, the helping professional operates with the clear-cut expectation and, indeed, the societal mandate that her or his efforts will make such a difference. Thus even if the practice of time-limited intervention has a reasonable body of evidence supportings its overall effectiveness, as Chapter 1 outlined, many specific questions still remain. For example:

- What are the actual procedures of the major approaches to short-term therapy as these *which* have been substantiated in empirical studies?
- How can an approach be altered to meet the particular characteristics of a given client or to adapt to some unique set of problem circumstances?
- How is client participation in the brief methods of therapy elicited and enhanced?
- What specific characteristics of technique and strategy differentiate brief methods of treatment from long-term intervention?
- What existing forces are already functioning in the lives of our clients that can be tapped as a part of the natural remedial process in order to augment the interventive process?

The accepted response to these and many similar issues has been to turn to theory of some kind—or to devise a new theory. As I pointed out earlier, there has been no lack of theoretical frameworks purporting to answer these central questions. In the face of the competing demands of so many viewpoints, it is all too easy for practitioners to simply resort to an uncomfortable mixture of theories and describe themselves as "eclectic." Jayarantne (1978) recently surveyed a large sample of clinical practitioners and found that 55 percent identified themselves as eclectic. A further 25 percent reported that they employed more than one theoretical framework and, under a broad definition, could also be considered eclectic. Among those self-identified as eclectic, nearly 20 percent reported the use of *five or more* conceptual frameworks in their practice. Other surveys have reported similar findings (Garfield and Kurtz, 1977).

The predominance of eclecticism among clinicians has been criticized, usually by those advocating strict adherence to a single theory (Greene, 1978; Wolpe, 1969). Yet there is little doubt that the front-line practitioner has scant opportunity to reflectively weigh the merits of a plethora of competing theories. The clinician is constantly confronted by the need to act and through action to promote positive change in clients who all too often do not neatly fit the cleaner categories of *any* theoretical framework.

In this chapter I will advance the thesis that no *one* theoretical framework is sufficiently comprehensive to meet the demands of short-term practice and that the helper must necessarily adopt some form of eclecticism. As the term "eclecticism" has gained a number of unfortunate connotations—suggesting a lack of choice, an unthinking mixing up of borrowed concepts, a Charlie-Brown-like wishy-washiness—I prefer to call this position "pluralism," although I am quite aware that what I am advocating is little different from what others have described as eclecticism.

Each of four major theoretical formulations will be discussed from several perspectives: (1) as a sort of distillation of the practice wisdom concerning the technical procedures of a substantiated method; (2) for clues to the management of the immediate interaction and relationship between helper and client while preparing for, or carrying out, an intervention; (3) as an avenue to developing a clearer understanding of the theoretical knowledge particularly related to short-term treatment, and (4) as a source of ideas about further change methods which might be utilized in short-term intervention.

THEORY AND PRACTICE

Practitioners easily become impatient with theory and tend, at times, to reject it out of hand as unrelated to the immediate necessities of practice. Yet no one can function without a "theory" of some sort, even if this is only the loosest collection of everyday notions about why people experience difficulties (or live successfully) and what they might do to overcome a problem in living. For example, Strupp (1978) studied the therapeutic effectiveness of laypersons without formal training in comparison with professionally trained therapists. He comments:

> On the other hand, a nonprofessional therapist may have a rationale, albeit commonsensical. For example, a college professor who functioned as an "alternative therapist" in the recent Vanderbilt project tended to insist that his patients (anxious, depressed and withdrawn male college students) suffered from "girl problems." He used this rationale quite effectively in his therapeutic interviews [p. 12 n.].

Turner (1974) offers one of the more perceptive analyses of the utilization of theory in the recent clinical literature. His discussion suggests multiple uses for theory, including the following: (1) a theoretical framework (whether singular or pluralistic) allows us to predict the outcomes of potential interventions; (2) theory helps to recognize unanticipated relationships between variables; (3) it assists us in identifying similarities or differences from one context to another and in realizing when there are deficits in our knowledge, and (4) finally, it serves as a baseline for assessing other theories. In addition, Turner notes that "theory gives assurance to the worker" (p. 13). In relation to this, he raises a provocative issue:

> We must have a set of anchoring concepts from which to work to avoid the aimless, albeit benevolent, wandering with the client that comes from lack of knowledge. Somewhat cynically, one might suggest that theory, whether it be sound theory or not, gives a sense of security to the therapist, thus increasing his certainty, thus increasing his effectiveness, even if what he does is not related to the theory he espouses. . . . A more telling and troubling question for me is whether at this stage in our practice development we need a theory except to serve as our anchor as mentioned above [p. 13].

I believe that this frank recognition of the pragmatic value of theory should be neither as troubling as Turner indicates nor, as he suggests later, "not a respectable question in a profession seeking increased recognition in the company of scholars" (p.

13). If it is the case, as the research evidence suggests, that all of the major theoretical orientations have developed interventions that are of roughly equivalent effectiveness (Bergin and Lambert, 1978; Frank, 1979; Garfield, 1980; Luborsky et al., 1975; Parloff, 1979; Strupp, 1978), then it is unlikely that any single one of these frameworks is, in an ultimate sense, the "correct" theory. Obviously all contain viewpoints that at least are sufficiently persuasive to the practitioner that some usable guidelines for practice can be derived. Perhaps most importantly, all offer the degree of assurance necessary to provide a sense of confidence in actual intervention.

Beyond these issues I believe that the clinical literature contains many highly useful ideas concerning the immediate application of the major methods that have received at least a reasonable degree of empirical substantiation. For example, many clinicians have written about the intricacies of developing an influential relationship with clients or the ways in which motivation can be enhanced so that it is possible to engage the client in the activities—verbal, emotional, or physical—that a given change method prescribes. It is one thing to know that assertive training, for instance, is useful with people who are encountering certain kinds of difficulties in their personal relationships but often an entirely different matter to induce the client to learn and employ these skills. Similarly, the clinician may have good reason to believe that careful, reflective examination of one's attitudes and values about close relationships may be helpful to a troubled individual, but it is much more difficult to persuade the client to actually engage in what may be an entirely unfamiliar process to that person.

Much of my consideration of the clinical literature, in the following sections, will be from this perspective. That is to say, I will not regard the generalizations of any theory as true or false in an absolute sense, but will attempt to probe their usefulness in this vital task of preparing, motivating, and supporting clients toward the successful utilization of the short-term helping process.

Social Learning Theory Influences

In his brilliant overview of the current status of social learning theory, Albert Bandura (1977b) points out that the most popular theories of human development and behavior have focused upon the individual and have emphasized such motivational forces as needs, drives, and impulses. Bandura believes that this approach to psychological theory is inadequate and is now being challenged, particularly by the comprehensive viewpoint contained in social learning theory.

In the social learning viewpoint an adequate explanation of behavior must include the antecedent inducements that may stimulate it, the expected benefits that it will produce, and, furthermore, such cognitive factors as "anticipations, intentions and self-evaluations" (Bandura, 1977b, p. 3.). It is in this latter area of cognitive factors, and their mediating and interpretive role in human function, that current social learning theory has significantly expanded upon previous behavioral theories. Thus from the social learning perspective there is no qualitative or etiological difference between prosocial or deviant behavior. The distinction is one of social norm or cultural evaluation, and all behaviors are viewed as acquired and maintained on the the basis of the same three regulatory systems. These will be briefly reviewed:

1. Certain human responses are primarily effected by external environmental events. For example, Pavlov's experiments demonstrated that the salivary responses of his dogs could come under the control of an external stimulus—in this case the ringing of a bell. On the other hand, external stimuli may less directly control behavior by virtue of their association with previously rewarding events. In this instance, the external stimulus acts as a *signal* to the individual that behaving in a particular way is likely to bring about reward or satisfaction. Thus recently developed weight reduction programs have enhanced their effectiveness by teaching the dieter to identify and deliberately alter the physical settings in which overeating had commonly occurred. By consistently reducing exposure to these previously stimulating circumstances, the

effect of other aspects of the program—reduced food intake, exercise, and so on—can be considerably enhanced.

2. A second major regulatory system lies in the feedback received, usually in the form of reinforcing consequences, for a behavior. *What* will be reinforcing, of course, is unique to each individual but may include satisfying experiences from the behavior itself (sexual orgasm, for example), tangible objects such as candy or money, or the person's own self-evaluative comments. In contrast to the stereotyped image of the behavior modifier as confined to doling out M and M's, many recent behavioral approaches have utilized this last reinforcement category. That is to say, clients have been taught to selectively increase their own rate of self-reinforcement as a potent change strategy. In any event, there is no doubt that consequences powerfully affect human functioning, both eliciting and maintaining behavior, and must be appropriately modified if change is to take place.

3. Finally, social learning theory has emphasized the influence of what Bandura (1977b) calls "central mediating processes" as the third, and perhaps most influential, regulatory system. These are the complex of cognitive processes through which human beings organize, codify, and symbolically store their daily experiences. Over time these cognitive factors become stabilized into attitudes, beliefs, and values and consequently play an essential part in governing behavior. The currently developing approaches in cognitive behavior therapy (Mahoney, 1974; Meichenbaum, 1974), for example, are designed to train clients in identifying and altering the cognitive patterns that may be operating to arouse unwanted and uncomfortable emotions or to inhibit or weaken desired behaviors. Chapter 9 will review the application of these, and other cognitively oriented approaches, to short-term treatment.

IMPLICATIONS FOR TREATMENT

Several other important guidelines for short-term intervention can be drawn from social learning theory in addition to the various change strategies noted above. These will be briefly reviewed here, but will be expanded upon in subsequent chapters of this book.

1. *The principle of specificity* suggests that learning takes place most efficiently when its target and goals are clearly and concretely identified by both therapist and client. This not only makes the process of change more readily apparent to both participants but also offers the client a modicum of protection against change efforts that he or she might not regard as desired.

2. *The principle of successive approximations* (or shaping) emphasizes that change takes place most easily in a series of steps or phases. A common frustration for disturbed individuals results from their thwarted attempts to change "at a blow," so to speak. Much of the skill of the therapist lies in an ability to break down a desired goal into its constituent elements or steps and to encourage the client in the systematic use of such a process.

3. *The principle of modeling* entails the finding that a great deal of complex human learning takes place through observing the behavior of others. Again, a part of the skill of the therapist lies in arranging and encouraging the use of needed modeling experiences. Therapists of many orientations have characterized the helper and the helping process as a type of modeling experience for the client. However, it must be remembered that modeling is a very literal process—what is observed is what is learned. If, for example, the client only observes the therapist asking questions or making brief, noncommittal replies, then it may be doubtful if any tangible skills for living can be learned from this example.

4. Finally, *the principle of performance* emphasizes that change takes place most readily when the individual tests out the new behavior through actual activity. Even such obviously cognitive factors as expectations or attitudes, as well as specific motor behaviors, are most significantly influenced in situations where the person can be induced to act (Bandura, 1977a; Bandura et al., 1980). This important principle underlies the stress placed in short-term treatment on such active change strategies as behavior rehearsal and task assignment.

Crisis Theory and Crisis Intervention

Perhaps because of its apparent simplicity, and undoubtedly because of its great utility, crisis theory and its practice counterpart of crisis intervention have been readily assimilated into the practice of most clinicians. In her critical review Lukton (1974) summarizes the most common formulation of the crisis state:

> . . . external and internal stimuli repeatedly produce stress, which in turn creates problem-solving situations for the individual. If the individual's usual means of problem solving do not work in a given situation, the result is called a crisis. Everyone possesses mechanisms for coping with stress that were developed in previous stress situations. Everyone goes through many crises in the course of living, and individuals may not be able to cope with specific crises. When an individual's coping mechanisms are unequal to solving the problems created by a stressor event, he will feel anxiety, and in this situation he will be in a state of active crisis [p. 386].

Crisis intervention, although still popular, was in particular vogue during the decade of the 1960s, and such writers as Lydia Rapoport (1970), Howard Parad (1965), and Gerald Caplan (1964) have extensively discussed its theory and practice. Others, such as Wittman (1961) and Meyer (1970), have gone so far as to propose that crisis intervention, based on an ecological framework, should become the major mode of social work service delivery, geared to serve the needs of a series of identifiable populations at risk.

The explanatory principles of the theory emphasize several key points:

1. Life is commonly characterized by any number of events, anticipated or unanticipated, which have the capacity to induce stress. Certain of these stress-inducing situations such as beginning school, entering adolescence, or getting married are almost inevitable happenings in the lives of most people. Others, such as

divorce, life-threatening illness, or disasters like hurricanes or earthquakes, are products of unique sets of circumstances. However, both the "normal" crises of unfolding life and the "situational" crises of unexpected events can induce acute stress in the vulnerable individual.

2. People vary in their ability to withstand or cope with stress. Whether any set of circumstances, normal or situational, induces a full-blown crisis state is a function of this individually determined capacity. However, it is important to note that the precipitating stimuli for crisis are not uncommon events, but are frequent enough in the life of anyone. Haley (1974), for example, has extended the notion of normal crisis in his discussion of the family life cycle. In this description of family living he points out how the progression from family of origin through courtship, marriage, the arrival of children, and so on, places increasingly complex demands upon the coping abilities of the family members. From this perspective many family problems can be seen as consequences of an accumulated crisis in living when the solutions that are functional in one stage of life become dysfunctional in a succeeding stage.

3. Once an individual has moved into crisis, a characteristic set of affective, cognitive, and behavioral manifestations are triggered that typify the crisis state. Although these reactions mimic many of the manifestations of emotionally disturbed or even psychotic individuals, crisis theory has emphasized that they are not pathological, but the expected and normal reactions to crisis. Indeed, Hansell (1973, 1975) has integrated crisis theory with the findings of social psychology and social anthropology to suggest that an individual's behaviors in crisis not only represent personal stress reactions but also serve as signals, to family and friends, of an urgent need for help.

4. Finally, both crisis theory and the practice of crisis intervention emphasize that the crisis state is temporary and, within a relatively short time, its acute characteristics will abate. It has usually been proposed that the actual crisis state persists for six to eight weeks, and consequently the need for rapid intervention has

been stressed.* This has been seen as necessary in order to intervene at a stage where the individual, because of heightened emotional discomfort, is most accessible to help. In addition, however, rapid intervention has been conceptualized as important in preventing the crisis victim from settling into a regressed and dysfunctional resolution of the crisis state.

TREATMENT STRATEGIES

Crisis intervention has developed a number of interventive strategies that have strongly influenced the practice of all forms of short-term treatment. As Rapoport (1970) has suggested, the treatment offered by the crisis worker must maintain a strong orientation to the present and, in order to emphasize this focus, is characterized by a deliberate use of such active and direct techniques as advice, suggestion, and education. All of this thrust is designed to restore the client to independent functioning within a relatively brief time period. Some clinicians have compared crisis intervention to the directive approaches successfully utilized with "school phobic" children and suggested that the central emphasis should be on a *rapid return to function.* For example, in the family crisis therapy described in some detail in Langsley and Kaplan's (1968) *The Treatment of Families in Crisis,* the crisis team give explicit tasks and assignments to the family in a planned effort to immediately stimulate at least the rudiments of social functioning.

Golan (1974) highlights some other distinctive features in her description of the initial contact in crisis intervention:

> The nature of the therapist/client relationship assumes a different form in crisis intervention, as in other forms of brief therapy. On

---

*A recent empirical study by Lewis et al. (1978) suggests that the duration of crisis, although still time-limited, may be somewhat longer than these commonly accepted limits. Their comparative examination of crisis in hospitalized patients found that such cognitive manifestations of stress as helplessness or lowered self-esteem persisted as long as twenty-seven weeks.

the one hand, the practitioner needs to establish quick rapport, both in order to elicit needed information quickly and to inspire confidence that he can help; on the other, the traditional concept of a ''meaningful relationship'' largely based on a leisurely exploration and testing over time and which often deepens into regressive transference, has little place in this form of treatment [p. 434].

A pervasive theme in almost all of the writings on crisis intervention is this emphasis on the active and direct role played by the therapist. Indeed, this theme is a common one throughout the entire family of brief therapies. Even the psychodynamically influenced short-term methods contain a similar stress, as the interview transcripts in the recent volume by Davenloo (1978) clearly illustrate. As neither activity nor directionality has especially characterized the conventional role of the helping person, much of the material in succeeding chapters of this book will attempt to illuminate this key aspect of short-term practice.

The Contribution of Ego Psychology

The major refinements in psychoanalytic thought fostered by such theorists as Anna Freud (1946), Erik Erikson (1950), Heinz Hartmann (1958), and David Rapaport (1967) have been variously characterized as ego-analysis or ego psychology. Although accepting many of the basic Freudian tenets regarding human behavior and development, ego psychology has been distinquished by its emphasis on the direct study of normal human functioning, its interest in the manner in which each individual develops a unique complex of ways of managing daily living, and, consequently, a stress upon social and environmental factors as ''powerful behavior elicitors and modifiers, above and beyond the psychological energies (drives)'' (Ford and Urban, 1963, p. 182). Ego psychology's detailed analysis of the conscious mechanisms of human functioning, particularly in relationship to the immediate environment, has profoundly influenced psychotherapeutic thought, and additionally is not incompatible with the more recent formulations of social learning theory.

In their attempts to expand existing psychoanalytic theory, the ego-analysts concentrated upon a careful examination of the functions of the ego, not simply as an arbitrating mechanism between the instinctual urgencies of id drives and the harsher strictures of the superego, but as a uniquely human capacity to understand and control one's life. Ford and Urban (1963) summarize this more optimistic viewpoint:

> The ego-analysts do not view man as an automaton pushed hither and yon by imperative energies on the one hand and by situational events on the other, constantly seeking some compromise among these conflicting influences. When behavior develops in a healthy fashion, man controls both it and the influence of situational events, selectively responding to seek consequences he has thoughtfully selected [pp. 187–188].

Thus human development must be conceptualized in relation to the emergence of the ego and its executive functions. This involves the central characteristics of consciousness (or attention) and the uniquely human capacity for thought, which act together, through the epochs of the life cycle, to refine and expand the individual's adaptation to his or her particular social context. Defense mechanisms, for example, not only serve as a means of avoiding or reducing anxiety but, in all of us, become the ingredients of personal style or character (Shapiro, 1965). These and the many other specific ego processes and functions are inherently neither good nor bad, but must be assessed in relation to the reciprocal demands of personal aspirations and societal expectation.

Briefly, ego psychology can be seen as highlighting three major themes of importance to the short-term practitioner:

1. Human growth (and, in general, personal development) takes place within a social context as an adaptive, purposeful process. In major respects this process is quite independent of the

instinctual energies postulated by orthodox psychoanalytic theory.

2. This patterned organization of the personality takes place not only through such specific devices as defense mechanisms but via the development and refinement of the human capacity for memory, anticipation, judgment, self-control, and, broadly speaking, personal character or style. All of this thrust, moreover, must be seen as in the service of living within, and coping with, the social environment.

3. Finally, ego psychology has stressed the detailed examination of normal human development, in this adaptive sense, beginning in infancy and early childhood but, importantly, continuing throughout later life epochs, each characterized by typical personal tasks and societal demands. All of this, as Maluccio (1979) has noted, highlights the person as actively coping with life and, within the helping encounter, as a significant participant rather than simply a recipient of service.

In this latter respect ego psychology has been especially influential in its identification of the important modifications in personality that take place, within the social context, throughout latency and adolescence and on into the various phases of adult life. Erikson's writing (1950) has delineated the adaptive demands in terms of a series of critical tasks, each representing a combination of personal value, societal norm, and coping necessity, broadly characteristic of each phase. The practice of short-term psychodynamic therapy, particularly in the approaches described by Mann (1973) and Sifneos (1972), has been heavily influenced by these formulations.

TREATMENT CONSIDERATIONS

An active cluster of therapists have contributed to the development of the short-term psychodynamic methods and, in this process, adapted many conventional techniques to the brief treatment model. James Mann (1973) identifies the five major techniques of suggestion, abreaction, manipulation, clarification, and interpretation, while Judd Marmor (1979) outlines a very similar group of strategies. Even practitioners who do not specifically utilize a psychodynamic base (or even reject these theoretical principles) are highly likely to employ some version of these techniques.

Suggestion. The therapist may give specific directives and advice to the client or, less directly, may embed suggestions within the overall framework of discussion with the client. Marmor (1979) points out that the persuasive influence of the clinician may also be compared to a process of operant conditioning in which "overt and/or covert indications of approval or disapproval from the therapist . . . move the patient in the direction of 'mental health' " (p. 153).

Abreaction. Within the safety of the therapeutic context (and relationship) the patient or client is encouraged to discharge strong emotions verbally and as Marmor (1979) suggests to "achieve a release of tension (catharsis) in a setting of hope and expectation of help" (p. 153).

Manipulation. From Mann's (1973) viewpoint this technique includes the multitude of direct or indirect ways in which the therapeutic alliance influences the client. It refers particularly to the corrective emotional experience that a positive and accepting relationship can provide. Marmor (1979) speaks of an "identification with the therapist in which the patient (usually unconsciously) models himself after the therapist" (p. 153). However, Marmor also notes that the treatment experience may involve "aspects of practice and rehearsal of new adaptive techniques and their generalization" (p. 153), and this emphasis on direct adaptive learning has, of course, many resemblances to the behaviorist's emphasis on the same area.

Clarification and interpretation. These techniques refer to two levels of intellectual or verbal intervention. In clarification, according to Mann (1973), the therapist's responses tend to pinpoint or summarize the significant emotional or interpersonal themes the patient is discussing. The usual goal is to impart greater specificity and emotional depth to these themes or, in other instances, to highlight connections or patterns that the client has not noticed. Interpretation, of course, is the uniquely psychodynamic technique of offering inferences based on the therapist's assessment of unconscious motivations or dynamic patterns in the client's life. Marmor (1979) subsumes both of these techniques under the heading of "cognitive learning" in apparent recognition of their intended purpose of bringing about change in the troubled person's attitudes, beliefs, or values.

Ego psychology has further implications, I believe, for any form of brief treatment in relation to its consistent focus upon the interaction between person and social environment. This dual focus on person and milieu can be clearly seen in Wasserman's (1974) discussion, from an ego psychology perspective, of a case vignette. He describes the following situation at the point of referral:

> Myron, age 12, black, was originally referred by the school because of his use of vile language, referring to the teacher as a "white bitch." He constantly chased other children, dragging them to the ground. Teacher and principal described mother as uncooperative, extremely hostile, "dangerous," insisting that the only recourse would be transferring Myron to an "adjustment" school. Mrs. M. disregarded all requests to come to the school, and with the Attendance Officer, Mrs. M. displayed an attitude of indifference followed by vulgar, abusive language. At one point, the Principal warned Mrs. M. that Myron could not graduate, that he was "crazy" and needed help. Mother was unhappy about this and agreed to talk to a social worker [pp. 60–61].

From this brief sketch Wasserman poses several questions that the therapist might will contemplate prior to entering this situation in a helping role. For example, he asks what it might mean to Myron, a black adolescent, to be taught by a white teacher. Similarly, he suggests that Mrs. M's reactions could be seen as efforts to cope with a school (and, in the interview with the principal, an immediate situation) that she, as a struggling single parent, perceived as attacking and unsympathetic. On the other hand, he suggests that the reactions of school personnel cannot be considered in isolation, but must be viewed as responsive to the threat they perceived in the behavior of mother and son. In these and other reflections, Wasserman illustrates the ego psychology theme of examining the adaptive (though not always successful) interaction between an individual and the impinging environment. The attempt is to illuminate such mutually determined responses, rather than to concentrate on either individual or environment alone.

Many of the postulates of ego psychology, developed during its heyday from approximately 1930 to 1950, are strikingly similar to the concepts advanced by Sullivan's (1953) interpersonal relationship theory and, most recently, by Albert Bandura's (1977b) integrative overview of social learning theory. For example, the ego-analysts' emphasis on social adaptation parallels the interpersonal relationship stress on the significance of familial and other intimate relationships. Similarly, there are startling resemblances between ego psychology's explication of such ego functions as self-control or stimulus nutriment (or, in general, the development of adaptive coping patterns) and the social learning theory emphasis upon very similar concepts.

Interpersonal Relationship and Family Theory

Like ego psychology, the principles of Harry Stack Sullivan's (1953, 1954) interpersonal relationship theory have profoundly influenced psychotherapeutic thought. But it would appear that the influence of the interpersonal relationship framework has assumed an even more covert and unacknowledged presence than ego psychology. Clinicians are often quite unaware of the impact of this conceptual framework on their practice. For example, a good deal of contemporary family and marital theory and practice has been strongly influenced by the interpersonal viewpoint. This is particularly evident in the highly popular communicational-interactional approach espoused by Haley (1963), Jackson (1965), and Satir (1964) and, in more recent years, refined and expanded by Salvador Minuchin and his co-workers (1967, 1974, 1978). All of these present-day approaches owe a heavy debt to Sullivan's earlier formulations.

The theoretical viewpoint that Sullivan developed is a psychology of people—their immediate effects upon one another and the critical role personal relationships play in forming and, furthermore, maintaining individual response. Indeed, for interpersonal relationship theory the notion of personality as an individual entity is truly an abstraction, a conceptual convenience. A person is not simply the product of prior experiences, but, within the flexible boundaries of her or his behavioral and emotional repertoire, is constantly shaped and influenced by the promises and demands of the personal environment.

Thus the interplay between the budding individual and the various people in his or her life is seen, not simply as a matter of adjustment or coping, but as formative of the essential patterns that we call personality. Moreover, this interpersonal influence continues through life, and, from a totally consistent interpersonal perspective, it would not be accurate to characterize a person as, for example, "suspicious" or "angry" as if this were a static or enduring aspect of character. Instead, one must specify the interpersonal situations in which these emotions occur— "suspicious when her employer praises her" or "angry when his wife is uninterested in sex."

The human organism must of course meet certain essential biological needs, but even these, in many respects, are qualified and mediated by interpersonal relationships. Uniquely human, however, is the capacity for anxiety, first experienced in relation to the mothering person but continuing throughout life in varying shapes and manifestations. Anxiety, in interpersonal relationship theory, is an experience between people, and the unit of analysis, in understanding any aspect of this phenomenon, must include at least two persons. More specifically, anxiety is the affective or emotional component of the perception that one's status with another person is diminished. This experience involves some degree of threat to self, and, as Sullivan (1954) points out, "any lowering of self-esteem is experienced as anxiety" (p. 96).

Yet at the same time that people experience anxiety in their immediate relationships with others there is also, in the absence of human intercourse, the powerful experience of loneliness. Sullivan (1954) postulated that loneliness, as the felt component of a lack of any close human relationship, was as potent a motivating force in personal interaction as the avoidance of anxiety. He makes a telling comparison between the two experiences:

> Under no conceivable circumstances has it ever occurred to me that anyone sought and valued the experience of anxiety. . . . No one wants to experience it. Only one other experience—that of loneliness—is in this special class of being totally unwanted [pp. 94–95].

A good deal of human interaction, then, involves a delicate balancing of the need to avoid anxiety and the need to reduce loneliness. Certainly one can entirely avoid anxiety, as it is transmitted through relationships with other people, by simply eliminating all personal contacts. But this solution, the hermit's choice, inexorably propels the individual into the countervailing experience of loneliness. It would be inaccurate, however, to convey the notion that interpersonal relationship theory pictures life as a precariously uncomfortable process of balancing anxiety and loneliness or as a painful series of choices between one or the other. Human relationships can also offer security, the felt experience of heightened self-esteem, and, through intimacy, the satisfying rewards of close personal association. These positive aspects of human intercourse can promote growth and satisfaction in any of us and at the same time enhance our ability to cope with the exigencies of life.

Finally, Sullivan (1953) traced out, in considerable detail, a series of stages in human life through which skill in interpersonal relationships is developed. Throughout this schema of development considerable emphasis is placed on the interpersonal context in which such learning takes place. Initially, of course, the child learns in relationship to the mother (or mothering person), but as life unfolds, increasingly complex and demanding social situations develop. More and more people play a part in the individual's life, and what we loosely refer to as "the environment" becomes increasingly populated.

TREATMENT CONSIDERATIONS

In its transition into the principles we now call "family theory," the interpersonal focus upon relationships among groups of people has singled out the family as a primary factor in both eliciting and relieving dysfunction. Thus family relationships can constitute a potent source of stress and anxiety. At the same time, the family can offer its members a highly meaningful refuge from the everyday pressures of living. The practitioners of family treatment have gone far beyond this simple position, of course, in developing a complex of theoretical statements concerning the processes governing family structure and interaction. From this has evolved a series of techniques and strategies for intervention with the family. All of this is far beyond the basic position of interpersonal relationship theory and will not be considered in this brief review. It will be sufficient to note that the family orientation of the interpersonal relationship framework— the belief that immediate family relationships can significantly affect individual behavior—has been a major influence in a number of brief interventive approaches. This influence is apparent whether or not the modality of treatment actually involves direct family interviews.

An example of this can be seen in the case of Mr. Antonini, whose pressing difficulties with ridicule and harassment from his co-workers were described in the first chapter of this book. The family orientation of the therapist played a significant role in the intervention. Initially this viewpoint influenced the clinician to invite both Mr. and Mrs. Antonini to the first session and see them together to discuss the difficulties Mr. Antonini was experiencing. The actual intervention involved work on sexual reeducation and assertion training for Mr. Antonini, and again both spouses were seen throughout the sessions. This approach was helpful, not because the focus was on marital conflict, but because Mr. Antonini, as a frightened, dispirited individual, needed all the effective support that could be mobilized at this critical point in his life. His wife was available and receptive to this role—a natural helping resource—and engaging her active participation also had the effect of demystifying the helping process and reducing much of the stigma her husband felt.

Perhaps the other major contribution of interpersonal relationship theory to short-term clinical practice lies in its emphasis on the therapist as both observer and participant in the helping process. From the very beginning of the therapeutic relationship the clinician must be aware of how he or she affects, and is affected by, this immediate interaction. This refers to much more than one's general level of awareness of attitudes toward certain types of people or one's overall values about such important issues in living as intimate relationships, child-rearing practices, divorce, abortion, and the like. The therapist and client, in this very immediate viewpoint, are inextricably caught up in a process of mutual influence within the interview situation. From the helper's side the very words that are employed, the phrasing or emphasis utilized in question or response, the gestures, voice tone, physical distance, and so on, all have their impact upon the client. The client's complex of behaviors has a similar effect upon the clinician, and these mutual reactions intertwine to form a process of reciprocal influence throughout a given session. Sullivan's (1954) perceptive analysis of the intricacies of therapeutic interviewing will be heavily utilized in the later discusssion of the management of the initial interview in short-term practice.

Commonalities among Theories

The several theoretical frameworks reviewed in this chapter have some distinct differences. Each posits a series of concepts to categorize and explain human behavior, or selected aspects of social functioning, and these terms certainly differ. There are obviously varied perspectives and philosophies influencing each theory. Comparatively speaking, some attempt to offer a panoramic explanation of human functioning, while others concentrate on only a selected aspect of the whole. Beyond these differences, I believe there are a number of common characteristics that are worth enumerating because of their immediate relevance to short-term intervention:

1. Theorists from each of these perspectives have been concerned primarily with explicating the major characteristics of *normal* human functioning as these unfold over the life cycle or are manifested under certain circumstances common to all human living. Thus there is a central emphasis on how people generally develop or respond to common life events rather than a focus on pathology per se.

2. All of the frameworks have suggested that the essential task of the individual is one of adaptation to the unique demands of his or her personal heritage—biological and cultural—and the immediate social milieu. The concept of adaptation, it should be noted, is an active one. It does not necessarily imply a passive acceptance of one's circumstances, but can include the possibility of highly creative response. Moreover, adaptation can also be seen as a *process* rather than a goal, and may include both successful and unsuccessful efforts.

3. This emphasis on adaptation, whether accepting or innovating, is especially appropriate to the task of the brief therapist. Many of the difficulties that come to the attention of members of the helping professions represent junctures where social adaptation has failed or where the individual's ability to cope has weakened. In other words, people seek help at the point where problems in living have developed. As a whole these theories offer the short-term clinician a comprehensive framework for understanding the places where functioning may typically falter, as well as potential guidelines for mobilizing constructive change efforts.

4. From each theoretical framework there is a heightened interest in the immediate activities of therapist and client within the helping process. Each of these participants is seen as an active agent in the change process, and, particularly in respect to the clinician's role, attempts to directly influence the client are viewed as not only helpful but unavoidable. The emphasis and value placed upon an active and immediate therapeutic role makes this cluster of conceptual frameworks especially suitable in articulating the process of short-term therapy.

5. Finally, the underlying philosophical stance of each of these theories suggests an optimistic view of humanity. Directly or implicitly each theory stresses the active interplay between person and environment that can foster the development of personal and social capacities. In each instance the individual is seen as playing an important governing role in his or her fate rather than as subject to uncontrollable forces, inner or outer. At the same time this optimistic viewpoint does not ignore or minimize the realistic threats and limitations to human attainment that can be contained in the environment or that may arise from unfortunate personal choices of the individual. Such a balanced emphasis between reality and optimism can be seen as central to the entire short-term treatment endeavor.

Chapter 3

Scenarios for Practice

Write the vision, and make it plain upon tables, so that a man may read it easily.

—Habakkuk, II, 2

Practitioners are often enough given an exposition of the theoretical principles underlying an approach to clinical practice, or descriptions of the research studies substantiating the effectiveness of a particular change strategy, but little notion of how the theory or empirical data are actually applied. This chapter will describe several typical short-term cases following the model outlined in the preceding chapters. Sufficient details will be given concerning the characteristics of the clients, their life problems, and the interventions employed that the practitioner will be able to form at least a rough cognitive map of the implementation of brief therapy. Many of the distinctive features of short-term intervention that these case descriptions highlight will be considered in greater depth in later chapters. The immediate objective is to give the clinician an overall view of the short-term treatment process in action.

Variations of Brief Treatment

The most important facets of the brief treatment model are the specificity of objectives, the emphasis on current problems in living, the frequent employment of structured change procedures, and the deliberate setting of a time limit for the intervention. Within these parameters, however, a number of variations are possible.

1. *Brief treatment within time limits.* The course of treatment may involve a designated number of interviews followed by termination of contact and, at the end of a planned time, a follow-up assessment. This, of course, is the basic model for brief therapy and perhaps its most common form. Its utility is suggested in the work of Gibbons and her colleagues (1979). These clinical researchers conducted a large-scale study in which task-centered casework, following Reid's model (Reid and Epstein, 1972), was offered to 200 persons following emergency hospitalization for a suicide attempt. They found that, for 54 percent of this group, time-limited intervention (averaging nine sessions) was both feasible and effective.

2. *Recontracting following an initial time-limited intervention.* It is possible that an additional period of contact must be negotiated at the usual termination point and intervention continued for a further time-limited period. This may occur where client and practitioner agree that goal achievement at the predicted termination point is insufficient and further work is needed. Recontracting may also be necessary in those instances where the client wishes to work upon a problem that was of lower priority at the initial contracting point but continues to be troublesome.

Gibbon's (1979) study of task-centered work with suicide attempters found that 17 percent were seen beyond the contracted time limits. The report does not say whether this extension of time involved continued work on the contracted problems or focus on another area of difficulty. However, it is interesting to note that this study reports a finding very close to that reported by Parad and Parad (1968) where 14 percent of their client population required extended treatment.

3. *Goal-oriented extended treatment.* In some instances therapist and client may decide that a series of interventions are

needed, each planned within explicit time limits and evaluated at the end of each segment. In this more extended type of contact there is still a high degree of goal specificity, and treatment does not continue from one segment to the next unless client and therapist agree that the projected objectives have been reasonably achieved and, furthermore, that continued help is needed. (Parenthetically it is worth briefly noting that if the goals for a given segment have not been achieved further treatment may be negotiated; if continued help is not needed intervention will terminate with, of course, a planned follow-up.)

4. *Periodic time-limited contact.* Finally, although many clients benefit from a single experience of short-term treatment, there are others who, for a variety of reasons, may need intermittent time-limited contact. Minuchin (1974, 1978) suggests that this approach to therapy is analogous to the conventional role of the family physician. Like the family doctor, the clinician provides continuous availability for brief periods of time to assist individuals with the normal (or unanticipated) difficulties of living.

Mrs. Altman, age 41, was initially seen for six sessions with the goal of deciding whether she should seek a divorce from her estranged husband. This was a particularly difficult decision for her to make because of her Middle Eastern cultural background, which had emphasized a subservient and submissive role for women.

She was seen eighteen months later and by this time had obtained a divorce and established herself in the teaching profession. However, she was fearful and guilty about resuming social and sexual relationships with men and was now seeking help with this difficulty. A twelve-session contract was negotiated.

There may be instances where certain characteristics of the treatment setting itself make this form of short-term intervention particularly useful. For example, in many inpatient or residential settings, although the client may by physically located within the institution for a lengthy period of time, continuous therapeutic service is not necessary over the entire stay. Instead of struggling to maintain a viable relationship during the periods when little movement is possible, both therapist and client can benefit from time-limited contacts at selected points. In many institutions contact will focus initially on the problems presented by the client's entry into the system and, later, by the difficulties encountered at reentry into the community. However, other difficulties may arise between these points where brief intervention can be feasible.

The first three of these variants will be illustrated in the case examples that follow. I will not offer any further exposition of the notion of periodic time-limited contact, as its principles are sufficiently similar to those of the other forms of short-term intervention that its implementation will be apparent.

Brief Treatment Within Time limits

Earlier I pointed out that surveys of clinical practice tend to substantiate that client contact in most instances is relatively brief and that truly lengthy treatment (whatever the intentions of the practitioner) is the exception. This suggests that much helping practice consists of *unplanned* brief treatment. Many of these brief contacts appear to involve a process in which helper and client work together for a certain number of sessions but without any agreed-upon time limit. Treatment terminates after several sessions, perhaps because the goals of intervention have been realized or, as often, because the client simply stops coming. Unless the client spontaneously returns for help at some later time, there is no further contact. This rather haphazard process is what many practitioners believe to be short-term treatment.

I have emphasized in the introductory chapter my conviction that this is an incomplete model for short-term therapy. Even in its most basic form, short-term helping should include both an explicit time limit for intervention and, after a designated interval, a planned follow-up session. Furthermore, the client should be aware that a follow-up session is planned and know its intended purpose, although I believe that the therapist should take the responsibility of arranging for the actual face-to-face interview.

Short-term intervention utilizing this basic model can be helpful in treating a wide variety of the personal, interpersonal, and social problems that concern many of the clients seen in such settings as family service agencies, mental health centers, general hospitals, and child guidance clinics. In conjunction with other modes of intervention the brief treatment model of engagement–intervention–follow-up can be utilized even in instances of severe dysfunction. Goldstein and his colleagues (Goldstein et al., 1978), for example, describe a six-session family-oriented approach, utilized with schizophrenics and their families, that was significantly effective in reducing relapse and rehospitalization rates. The brief therapeutic intervention was highly structured and heavily oriented toward the realistic social pressures commonly faced by ex-mental patients and their families. A sequence of closely related objectives were emphasized:

(1) The patient and his family are able to accept the fact that he has had a psychosis, (2) they are willing to identify some of the probable precipitating stresses in his life at the time the psychosis occurred, (3) they attempt to generalize from that to identification of future stresses to which the patient and his family are likely to be vulnerable, and (4) they attempt to do some planning on how to minimize or avoid these future stresses. [p. 1170].

In this study, it should be noted, the brief intervention was initiated at discharge from the hospital and combined with administration of the appropriate psychotropic medication to the schizophrenic family member.

The following cases are drawn from family service and mental health settings. Both illustrate the willingness of the helper to establish a helping contract in an area of the client's choosing and, further, to design an intervention that would specifically address this area of major concern—and no more. In other words, the therapeutic ambitions of the helper were disciplined by the limits defined by the clients.

CASE ILLUSTRATION: CONTROLLING ANGER

A physically handicapped, mildly retarded man in his late thir-ties, Mr. Jurecko reluctantly approached a family service agency for help with the temper outbursts toward co-workers that were jeopardizing his job in a large industrial firm. Both sensitive to his limitations and highly conscientious in his work, he had be-come increasingly vulnerable to the rowdy give-and-take of the working world. Mr. Jurecko's employer had stipulated that he must "get counseling" or risk losing his job.

It would have been all too easy to become overly absorbed in the implicit array of psychological, social, physical, and emo-tional complications suggested by even this sketchy vignette of Mr. Jurecko and his difficulties. The essence of helping, as Rab-kin (1977) emphasizes, lay in responding to Mr. Jurecko's re-quest for some immediately usable ways of controlling his temper, thus meeting his employer's concerns and, most impor-tantly, preserving his job.

It was apparent during the initial interview that Mr. Jurecko's difficulties on the job were arising from a number of sources. He had a moderately impairing handicap which placed some restric-tion on his physical capacities and made his speech heavily slur-red and difficult to understand. His education had been mainly in "special class" settings in the public school system and had given him only the most rudimentary of academic skills. Even after several attempts at vocational training (sponsored by various rehabilitation agencies) he had not been able to gain any market-able technical skill.

He took his job as operator of a freight elevator very seriously and showed an almost fierce pride in his reliable and responsible performance of his duties. In the insensitive atmosphere of the working-class world he sometimes encountered teasing and de-precating remarks from his fellow workers. This rough bantering created some stress, but additionally he described himself as often becoming extremely upset over what he viewed as the lazy and slipshod work attitudes of certain of his co-workers. Brief behavior rehearsals during the initial interview suggested that Mr. Jurecko possessed reasonably adequate assertive ability in situations where tension had not risen to too high a level. However, tension had been building over many months, and the two angry incidents which had precipitated his referral occurred on days when his dissatisfaction with himself, his job, and his co-workers had become particularly acute.

In both of these episodes Mr. Jurecko had become verbally abusive and shouted threats at other employees, and in one instance he had thrown a heavy piece of equipment across the room. Mr. Jurecko was realistically afraid that he might lose his job if he was not able to convince the management of the firm that he could control his temper in the future. He expressed discouragement about his handicaps and the restrictions they placed upon him but viewed them as limitations within which he had learned to live.

A contract was negotiated with Mr. Jurecko to concentrate on developing workable methods of temper control, and the therapist suggested that this goal was manageable within six sessions. It was explained to him that his angry outbursts could be seen as accumulated reactions to the stress he was encountering on a daily basis. This rationale was discussed with him and illustrated through references to the various situational and attitudinal factors he had described. He was told that the method of intervention would involve teaching him several ways of reducing stress in order to keep it from building up to unmanageable proportions. He was also informed that this approach would require that he practice the stress management techniques at home so as to gain proficiency, test them out and refine them in the actual work setting, and, finally, keep a daily record of tension-producing situations in order to follow his progress.

Intervention utilized an adaptation of the stress management model developed by Meichenbaum (1975) and, following these guidelines, emphasized (1) the development of behavioral skills in relaxation, and (2) attention to any cognitive cues that were engendering tension. Relaxation techniques involving muscular release and deep breathing were taught during the first three sessions, and Mr. Jurecko practiced these daily at home. He was asked to keep a very simple diary noting the occurrence and nature of any troublesome incidents at work.

The clinician's overall strategy was to provide Mr. Jurecko as quickly as possible with some tangible methods of reducing stress. It was felt that once his general tension level was diminished, he would be better able to look at how some of his own attitudes might be contributing to his stress. Perhaps fortuitously a minor incident came up on his job during the second week of treatment. As this situation was not too demanding, Mr. Jurecko was able to handle the pressures quite well, and this bolstered his confidence in himself and, implicitly, in the treatment approach. Fortified by his developing skills and this beginning success, he coped with some further difficult incidents over the following week with equal aplomb.

Work on stress reduction techniques continued over the final three weeks of the contact. This focused particularly on developing such key words as "relax" or "calm" as relaxation signals that could be utilized unobtrusively in public situations. In these final sessions the focus also incorporated general discussion of the realistic pressures of factory work. Additionally, Mr. Jurecko's demands upon himself to perform, as well as his feeling of being trapped in a dead-end job, were identified as factors contributing to his general level of stress. Within the context of short-term treatment the therapist's effort was to make Mr. Jurecko more aware of the impact of his own attitudes upon his difficulties rather than to resolve them.

A follow-up session with Mr. Jurecko three months later found him coping well with the day-by-day pressures of his job. He described a few episodes that had been upsetting to him, but he had been able to handle each of these without any undue outburst of anger. Although he was not using the stress management techniques consistently, it was apparent that he was able to call upon them as needed to reduce or control immediate tensions.*

CASE ILLUSTRATION: LEAVING HOME

In some instances the therapist may employ a straightforward problem-solving model in short-term intervention. The following case example, drawn from a community mental health setting, will illustrate the adaptation of this ''commonsense'' approach to therapeutic practice.

Mrs. Lorenson, a woman in her late twenties, was referred to counseling by a friend who had noticed her increasing preoccupation and apparent depression. She pictured herself in the initial interview as considerably upset about difficulties in two major areas of her life but unable to come to grips with either of these problems.

First, she had married about a year earlier, and, following a short honeymoon, her husband had been posted overseas by the multinational corporation by which he was employed. For various realistic reasons it had not been possible for Mrs. Lorenson to accompany him on the assignment. Throughout this enforced separation Mrs. Lorenson had been experiencing many misgivings about her marriage, which had been preceded by only a brief courtship, yet felt guilty and troubled about harboring such thoughts. Second, she was continuing to live at home with her elderly parents despite having quite adequate income to live elsewhere. Mrs. Lorenson was fearful of offending her parents by suggesting that she would feel happier and more comfortable in her own apartment.

Discussion and exploration of these two problems occupied the

*A chance encounter with Mr. Jurecko three years later provided further follow-up data. At that time he volunteered that he was maintaining his job without any major difficulty and was still using the tension reduction procedures at appropriate moments.

greater part of the first interview. Although her uncertainties about her marriage were most pressing and were causing the greater portion of her unhappiness, Mrs. Lorenson did not believe that she could reach any resolution of these feelings as long as her husband was out of the country. Until he returned and she could directly experience the relationship again, Mrs. Lorenson did not feel she could arrive at a realistic solution. On the other hand, despite its secondary status, her discontent with continuing to live at home was sufficiently strong that she wanted to do something about this quandary. It was agreed that six to eight sessions would be spent working on this problem.

The therapist followed a very simple problem-solving model over the sessions that followed. This model (D'Zurilla and Goldfried, 1971; Goldfried and Goldfried, 1975) suggests that once a problem is specifically identified, the first (and most critical) step is to translate it into a description of a desired goal. The goal statement may be thought of as a statement of how the client would want to be feeling, thinking, or acting if he or she no longer had the problem. In this case Mrs. Lorenson's problem of being discontented with living at home was transformed into the goal of moving into an apartment of her own. Other goals, such as gaining an understanding of why she was so deferential toward her parents, learning how she might live more comfortably in the parental home, or even the objective of moving to an entirely different city, might have been negotiated, but this was the goal that was most meaningful to Mrs. Lorenson. Achieving it became the purpose of counseling.

After the problem and goal statements have been sufficiently specified, then the problem-solving model stipulates that the necessary changes, leading from problem state to goal achievement, must be identified. These are usually visualized as a series of steps, or consecutive tasks, that will enable the client to progress from the present problematic situation toward the selected goal. Where the goal involves developing such social skills as assertive behavior, improved sexual functioning, or interpersonal communication, there may be a validated procedure in the clinical literature. Where this is the case, the function of the therapist would be to identify this change procedure, explain its expectations and limitations, and guide the client through the intricacies of its process. With many life situations, however, a unique series of steps need to be generated.

Brainstorming was used as a method of identifying the various steps that Mrs. Lorenson needed to take to reach her goal of independent living. In the brainstorming process both client and helper attempt to identify, in as imaginative and uncensored a way as possible, all of the elements that might be involved in moving toward the desired goal. Once a list of many such potential components has been generated, it is possible to eliminate the unfeasible or unnecessary steps and to arrange the remainder into a sequence leading to the desired goal. With Mrs. Lorenson the major steps included:

1. Decision making about the type, cost, and location of a suitable apartment
2. Searching for such accommodation through newspaper advertisements and real estate firms
3. Selecting an apartment and signing a lease
4. Informing her parents of her decision to move
5. Making the physical arrangements for the actual move

During the intervention all of these steps were more specifically defined, where necessary broken into component parts, and accompanied by pertinent task assignments. Arranging the steps of the implementation phase in a suitable progression may at times require some sensitivity and skill. The needed sequence of steps can be seen as following either a *logical* or an *emotional* hierarchy or, in some cases, aspects of both these. In the problem-solving intervention with Mrs. Lorenson both logical and emotional considerations were utilized.

The logical hierarchy is based on the notion that a complex goal can be broken down into a series of simpler elements, each of which in turn will contribute to the ultimate attainment of the desired goal. In job finding, for example, assessing one's strengths, skills, and relevant experience is almost always a necessary beginning point in the sequence. Thus in Mrs. Lorenson's case it was necessary to decide where she wanted to live and to determine whether suitable apartments were available in this area before further steps could be taken.

The concept of an emotional hierarchy recognizes that certain steps in a goal attainment sequence are more anxiety-provoking than others, and attempts to place the less fearful steps at the beginning of the implementation process. In assertion training, for example, the earliest steps are usually concerned with relatively simple assertions in the context of relationships of only minor emotional significance to the trainee. It is usually much less anxiety-provoking to deal with a clerk in a department store than to be assertive toward one's supervisor or spouse. Thus in work with Mrs. Lorenson one aspect of the problem-solving sequence was deliberately placed further into the sequence in order to avoid her having to confront an emotionally demanding step too soon. Specifically, Mrs. Lorenson might have informed her parents of her decision to move as an initial step in the problem-solving sequence. However, this step, at the therapist's suggestion, was not undertaken until several other steps had been accomplished. Mastering these easier tasks first not only increased Mrs. Lorenson's confidence in herself but also had the effect of increasing her sense of commitment to her goal before she even approached her parents.

The necessary steps in the problem-solving process were clearly identified within an interview or two, and by the sixth session Mrs. Lorenson was concluding arrangements to move into her own apartment. Homework assignments in the earlier phases had been helpful in mobilizing and focusing her energies, and some brief behavior rehearsal had prepared her for the step of informing her parents of the move. Like many feared encounters this latter task was managed relatively easily, with Mrs. Lorenson's parents showing little of the emotional upset she had anticipated.

At a follow-up interview a few months later Mrs. Lorenson was comfortably settled in her new apartment, and her relationship with her parents continued to be amicable. She had still had no opportunity to confront her misgivings about her marriage and looked forward to her husband's eventual return to the country with some understandable apprehension.

TREATMENT CONSIDERATIONS

Aside from following the general engagement–intervention–follow-up paradigm, both of these case illustrations incorporate a number of features typical of short-term treatment that are worth reviewing:

1. The focus of intervention was on directly responding to the immediate request of the client. In one instance this request was concerned with reducing the danger of losing a job; in the other illustration the client's concern was to be relieved of the discomfort of an undesired living situation. Although neither of these goals called for profound changes in the client, it was apparent that for both individuals a genuine problem existed that was beyond their immediate coping abilities.

2. Therapeutic intervention was designed to impact directly upon this request. A specific change method (stress management training) was utilized with Mr. Jurecko, while a more general problem-solving procedure was employed with Mrs. Lorenson. The clinician's responsibility was to identify an appropriate change strategy, guide and motivate the client in its application, and, as needed, assist in its adaptation to the particular needs of the client.

3. Although there were other areas of difficulty evident with both clients, the therapist did not attempt to intervene in these aspects of their lives. Mrs. Lorenson was quite clear that she did not believe she could resolve her doubts about her marriage until she had the opportunity for face-to-face discussion with her husband. Mr. Jurecko was less explicit about the other problems he was experiencing, but as the initial exploration revealed that his

most heightened concern was about the possibility of losing his job, the therapist concentrated attention upon this expressed difficulty.

There may be times when another problem directly interferes with or prevents resolution of the targeted problem. In such cases it is obviously the therapist's prerogative to point out this connection to the client, and work on the client's request may only be possible in conjunction with attention to this related difficulty. Clinicians should be cautious, however, in too quickly concluding that other considerations, of whatever theoretical variety, will block problem resolution. It should be remembered that a broad implication of the empirical evidence for the effectiveness of brief intervention is the strong suggestion that many difficulties can indeed be satisfactorily resolved despite the existence of concurrent problems in other aspects of the client's functioning. Thus the belief that understanding must be attained before behavior can be altered or that certain behaviors represent "symptoms" of deeper-seated difficulties, and so on, may be more a purely theoretical conviction than a compelling reason to defer attempts to induce specific change.

4. Finally, in both cases the therapist demonstrated a willingness to terminate work with the client at the projected ending point rather than look for reasons to continue. Haley (1967) identifies what he calls the "willingness to release patients" as a predominant characteristic of the provocative approaches to brief therapy practiced by Milton Erickson. He makes the following comments in relation to this aspect of Erickson's work:

> The framework he establishes in the therapeutic relationship has built into it the idea that the relationship is temporary to achieve particular ends. . . . Because of his positive view and his respect for patients, Erickson is willing to start a change and then release the patient to let the change develop further. He does not allow the needs of the treatment setting to perpetuate the patient's distress, as can happen in long term therapy. Since he does not see therapy as a total clearance, or cure, of all the patient's present and future problems, he is willing to give patients up. His approach is to

remove the obstacles which, once removed, allow the patient to develop his career in his own way [pp. 541–542].

As I shall point out, later in this chapter, the decision to terminate can sometimes be difficult, particularly if the client has not clearly achieved the goal of the intervention. However, the follow-up session offers some safeguard against the dangers of "abandoning" a client who still needs help. This consideration underscores the necessity of a planned follow-up contact and, furthermore, the need for the practitioner to be particularly conscientious in arranging this interview at its appropriate time.

Recontracting Following an Initial Intervention

The short-term therapist may find it necessary in certain cases to renegotiate the length of the intervention. A rough guideline, based on the data from the Gibbons et al. (1979) and Parad and Parad (1968) studies cited earlier as well as on my own clinical experience, suggests that this contingency may arise in perhaps one of every five or six short-term cases. The need for further time may become apparent at the termination session of the original series of sessions or at the follow-up interview. In either case, the decision to continue (or to extend the original contract) should be a mutual agreement between helper and client and, most importantly, based upon clear indications that the goals of intervention have not been reached. Alternatively, it is sometimes possible to find that the immediate intervention, though quite successful, has revealed a need to work upon another area of difficulty.

Case Illustration: Coping with Sexual Fears

Recurrent chest pains had impelled a twenty-six-year-old unmarried man, Dennis Faber, to visit several physicians and hospital outpatient clinics. Following the fifth such consultation, which had confirmed the previous findings that there was no physical basis for his pains, Mr. Faber was referred to a family service agency for counseling.

He was a friendly, talkative young man, somewhat disheveled in appearance, who anxiously described a series of immediate difficulties in his life. A high school graduate with some sporadic technical training, he had recently been fired from his job (for "inattention") and was considering going into business for himself as a TV and radio repairman. He was excited about this prospect but apprehensive as he had few financial resources except his unemployment compensation benefits and a battered old car.

At the same time, he felt dissatisfied and discouraged about his social relationships, particularly with women. Mr. Faber seldom dated, described himself as awkward and clumsy in even casual conversation with women, and was especially depressed about his lack of sexual experience. He saw himself as a sexual failure. Much of his difficulty, he believed, was due to his parents' extremely moralistic and inhibiting views in regard to dating and sexuality.

The initial interview with Mr. Faber was complicated by his voluble and anxious manner—he was an almost nonstop talker. Although a high degree of concern about his social and sexual competency was readily apparent, it was difficult to arrive at a definite contract to work upon this area. Rather than move ahead into treatment without a firm agreement about its goals, the therapist is well advised in such situations to arrange only a minimal contract entailing further problem exploration. In this case the helper suggested that one or two further sessions could be spent in considering how therapy might be most helpful to Mr. Faber.

These interviews were spent in exploring the several areas described above, and by the third session a positive agreement had been negotiated to work on increasing Mr. Faber's comfort and ability in social and sexual relationships with women. A time limit of ten to twelve sessions was stipulated by the therapist, and Mr. Faber was given some material on human sexuality to read (selected chapters from James McCary's [1973] *Human Sexuality: A Brief Edition*) as his first task.

The first six sessions with Mr. Faber had two major purposes. One objective was to assess his social skill level in heterosexual relationships and, if necessary, employ systematic behavioral training to increase his facility in this area. The other major goal was to reduce his obvious anxiety about sexuality. In the initial interviews he had shown a great deal of discomfort and embarrassment about even discussing sex, and it was quite apparent that his prudish and moralistic family background had significantly contributed to this difficulty. However, the approach to inducing change in this area was not historical. A variation of cognitive restructuring was employed in which reading assignments on sexual matters increased his factual knowledge. Simultaneously, direct discussion of his immediate doubts and curiosity, in the accepting atmosphere of the therapeutic relationship, consolidated this new knowledge and alleviated many of his concerns.

Training in heterosexual skills proved necessary. This training was not as basic as some socially awkward individuals require but did include important work on such areas as initiating conversations, asking for dates, expressing feelings and, broadly speaking, ways of developing a personal and potentially intimate relationship with women. In addition, some direct discussion on how to improve and maintain his personal appearance and hygiene was necessary. (These training methods are described in more detail in Chapter 8 on social skills.) During this period the interviews were typically divided between social skill training (and the behavior rehearsal methods used in its implementation) and more general reflective discussion of his reactions to the reading assignments on sexuality.

During the final six weeks of contact Mr. Faber's confidence in himself had increased sufficiently that the therapist encouraged him to begin active dating. He began rather hesitantly but within a few weeks had successfully managed to take out several young women. Although he felt awkward at times, he was pleased to find that the women he dated seemed quite satisfied with his company. As one might expect, the dates involved some of the kissing and fondling typical of beginning relationships and, on one occasion, sexual intercourse. These personal and sexual experiences provided further opportunity to refine the social skills developed in the earlier sessions and to support Mr. Faber's growing realization that he could be quite attractive to women.

Although Mr. Faber's experience was still limited, it appeared reasonable at the twelfth session to strongly emphasize his positive gains and to terminate active intervention. The therapist arranged to contact him for a follow-up session in three to four months. The decision to terminate at this point, rather than negotiate an extension of treatment, was influenced by the practitioner's conviction that Mr. Faber was moving forward in a positive way. It is often better to encourage this type of independent growth, by the very act of termination, than to foster uncertainty or dependency by continuing treatment.

The follow-up session, however, proved this clinical judgment to be wrong, as Mr. Faber was quite discouraged and bogged down. He had dated only sporadically since last seen and had lost most of the self-confidence that he had developed earlier. Mr. Faber felt baffled by his lack of progress, and a further series of sessions was negotiated. The therapist suggested that this second contact should be limited to eight sessions and should concentrate on remedying whatever was impeding Mr. Faber in utilizing his previously developed skills.

As there was good evidence that Mr. Faber's heterosexual skills were now adequate and that in general he was less anxious about sexuality, this continued intervention was much more cognitively oriented. Early exploration, both in the interview and through task assignment, attempted to identify any motivational or attitudinal factors that might be operative. Exploration of his self-dialogues when he was in the company of women suggested that certain of Mr. Faber's own expectations and beliefs were setting him up for failure. In addition, these same factors were creating considerable internal stress during any dating situation. For example, as he approached an attractive young woman, he often found himself thinking "She won't want to talk to me" or "She'll laugh in my face if I ask her for a date." Similar ruminations were affecting him during the course of a date. Some of these cognitive cues were identified by asking him to imagine himself in conversation with a woman. Others became apparent as he kept a daily log of his reactions.

As this mixture of self-deprecation and internally stimulated anxiety became evident, the difficulty Mr. Faber was meeting in utilizing the skill learning from the previous sessions became understandable. The therapist thereupon initiated training in cognitively oriented self-management methods, emphasizing to Mr. Faber that this would give him an active means of coping with the anxieties and uncertainties he was experiencing. It was pointed out, however, that self-management techniques of this sort would have little effect unless he deliberately employed them in the appropriate situations. In large part the first three sessions were devoted to basic relaxation training and, following the clinical guidelines suggested by Mahoney (1974), Meichenbaum (1975), and others, guiding Mr. Faber in learning how to use cue words and unobtrusive physical techniques in stressful situations. Homework assignments during this phase concentrated on practicing these techniques and refining their application in real life. Additionally, he was asked to mentally rehearse successful encounters with women in order to check his prevalent tendency to dwell upon negative anticipations.

This cognitive behavioral approach was helpful in offering Mr. Faber some tangible ways of managing himself but was not sufficient in stimulating him to move forward again. For two or three weeks he remained blocked and found various reasons to defer any serious attempts at resuming dating. He spoke of how busy he was in developing his new business and found minor flaws in all the women he met. The therapist attempted to respond to the genuine anxiety that was implicit in this impasse but by the sixth of the eight sessions decided that Mr. Faber must be confronted with the need to act, despite his fears. The confrontation had the desired effect of energizing Mr. Faber, and through the final weeks of counseling he began dating relationships with two women he had recently met. A good level of emotional comfort and social ease was evident in both these relationships, and active treatment was concluded at the eighth session.

A formal follow-up interview with Mr. Faber was delayed by vacation schedules and other contingencies until almost seven months after this final session. Telephone contact, however, had affirmed that he was quite satisfied with his social life and experiencing no obvious difficulties. This picture was even more positive when he was seen in a face-to-face follow-up session. By this time he was dating frequently and in the previous two or three months had become quite close to one young woman. They were enjoying a regular sexual relationship, and Mr. Faber no longer saw himself as the sexual failure he had once described. As a matter of fact, he was mildly perturbed by his girlfriend's hints that they should begin thinking of marriage or at least start living together. Although Mr. Faber did not think he was ready for marriage, he was also aware of the irony in now having to face an issue that had never confronted him as a ''sexual failure.''

SOME GENERALIZATIONS

Many of the same factors that characterized the two cases described earlier are also evident in the case of Mr. Faber.

1. Again it is evident that the practitioner of brief therapy takes an active and direct role in the *process* of specifying the major problems and goals of treatment, although the *content* of these goals is largely governed by the wishes of the client. That is to say, the therapist's insistence is upon the necessity of arriving at clearly understood objectives before beginning intervention, not upon the nature of these goals.

2. The course of treatment with Mr. Faber also demonstrates the short-term therapist's propensity for utilizing structured

change methods in which a sequence of steps or stages guide both helper and client activity. Although stress management techniques played a part in therapy with Mr. Faber, as with Mr. Jurecko earlier, this similarity is coincidental. The strategy of change could easily have been assertion training or some other structured technique if this had been responsive to the client's needs.

3. The work with Mr. Faber over the course of the two segments of treatment additionally illustrates the frequent need for a *package* of interventions. At various points not only stress management but social skill training and cognitive restructuring methods were combined with more conventional reflective discussion methods. The art of therapy often lies not only in the knowledgeable selection of a cluster of strategies but in their skillful integration in actual practice. My intent, however, is not to advocate a shotgun-like blast of technological virtuosity, but a sensitive adaptation of disparate inducements to change.

4. It will also be evident that brief therapy frequently takes a very literal approach to bringing about change in the client's daily life. Such an approach can seem almost embarrassingly direct and in many instances may involve nothing more or less than a concentrated effort to increase the activities or behaviors that will constitute goal attainment for the client. Thus when Mr. Faber wished to date more often, the most straightforward approach to this goal was to teach him the interpersonal skills most likely to increase his chances of obtaining dates with women. Once these skills became established, then the therapist became as direct in encouraging him to use them. Indeed, in the second segment of contact the therapist did not hesitate to confront Mr. Faber with the need for action.

5. At the same time, it would be inaccurate to suggest that short-term therapy is little more than a routinized and insensitive application of mechanical procedures. As I will discuss later at some length, the influence of the therapist is possible and meaningful only within the context of a warm and emotionally responsive relationship. In addition, carefully graduated task assign-

ments, consistent reinforcement and support, and watchful attention to adverse client reactions all play an integral part in the management of any change process, structured or otherwise.

6. Finally, throughout the intervention the therapist is alert to the immediate effects of the helping process. Are the strategies employed enabling the client to progress toward his or her desired goals? This does not necessarily require elaborate testing or monitoring devices, but in large part is managed through two features of brief intervention: First, the frequent tasks carried out by clients serve as probes, not only of their capacity and willingness to change but of the direction this change is taking. Second, the goals of intervention should be so clearly defined in the initial phase of contact that it will be quite apparent when they have been met or at least reasonably approximated. As I will discuss in Chapter 7 on tasks and homework, clients may be asked to keep diaries or charts which record aspects of their daily life, but these are more in the nature of information-gathering devices than precise evaluative instruments.

Goal-oriented Extended Treatment

There is no doubt that there are times when it is necessary, in the considered judgment of the clinician, to work with a client over a period of time that falls beyond the usual three- to fifteen-session boundaries of short-term treatment. This contingency may arise at the beginning of therapy, or it may become apparent after a brief intervention has proved unsuccessful. In such instances it is possible to adapt a number of the guiding principles of short-term intervention to the lengthier treatment. The extended contact can be broken down, for example, into a series of time-limited periods each of which concentrates on an identified problem or on a major component of the overall goal of treatment. Within these stages structured techniques can be used, client participation encouraged, and various devices utilized to evaluate the process of change. A case from a family service agency will illustrate this approach.

CASE ILLUSTRATION: BECOMING UNCOUPLED

Unlike many other conflicted couples, Mr. and Mrs. Toman entered marriage counseling at the instigation of the husband. They were a rather unexceptional lower-middle-class couple, both high school–educated. Mrs. Toman was now training as a medical technician at the local community college, while Mr. Toman worked at a minor clerical job in a large manufacturing firm. Both were in their late forties, and they had been married for more than twenty-five years. Although they had never been especially happy together, the past several years had been markedly difficult. Their two oldest children were now adults and on their own, while the two younger children were in college and, through scholarships, loans, and part-time work, essentially independent. Mr. and Mrs. Toman were finding themselves confronted with a decision about whether to continue a chronically dissatisfying marriage now that family responsibilities no longer bound them together.

Mrs. Toman described her husband as having been both dominating and unloving throughout their marriage and felt she had continued in the relationship only in order to provide a home for the children. Mr. Toman acknowledged many of the difficulties his wife recounted and agreed that he had been responsible for much of their estrangement. However, he thought that the problems had been exacerbated by the two serious heart attacks he had sustained about seven years earlier. Moreover, he was highly concerned to maintain the marriage as, from his strongly religious perspective, neither separation nor divorce was a viable alternative.

A six-session contract to explore the marital relationship and determine if it could be strengthened was agreed upon by both Mr. and Mrs. Toman. However, even at this early stage Mrs. Toman was a reluctant participant, and her reluctance became even clearer as the sessions proceeded. The tasks typical of short-term treatment served to highlight her almost total emotional disengagement from her husband, as she either did not carry them out or did so in only the most perfunctory manner.

Within three or four weeks it was apparent that there was little possibility of fruitful marriage counseling. The therapist utilized the remaining time, in both individual and conjoint sessions, to confront the couple with this bleak predicament.

The sixth session brought out Mrs. Toman's firm conviction that the marriage was utterly hopeless. She was only deferring divorce proceedings until she finished her technical training and could become self-supporting. This abrupt termination of marriage counseling and the prospect of a lengthy marriage coming to an end were a considerable shock to Mr. Toman. Hearing his wife speak so bluntly of her intention to divorce him evoked a great deal of immediate emotional turmoil. He readily accepted the therapist's offer of individual counseling. Mrs. Toman was not interested in any individual contact as she had a counselor, whom she had seen a year or two earlier, to whom she could turn.

The intervention with Mr. Toman continued over the next twelve months and involved more than forty interviews. It was not visualized as an extended contact at the beginning of treatment but evolved into this form as the evaluative work at the end of each segment indicated a strong need to continue counseling. It will be described in relation to the several goal-oriented phases, each of about eight to ten weeks' duration, into which it fell.

Dealing with crisis. Although he had been quite aware for several years that his marriage was failing, it was still a distinct shock to Mr. Toman to hear his wife openly declare her intention to divorce him. The fact that this had been not been said in the heat of a quarrel but announced in the relative calm of the final conjoint session added to its impact. A confusing welter of feelings and thoughts fueled his sense of crisis.

Initially, he felt strong anxiety about what his life would be like outside the familiar confines of even an unsatisfactory marriage. At the same time he was experiencing periodic surges of the almost formless but potent anger that grips one who must grapple with the realization that a central relationship has failed. These strong feelings were combined with a pervading sense of guilt stemming from his religious convictions and, at a less easily verbalized level, fear about his physical health and the possibility of further serious illness. This latter apprehension was by no means unrealistic. Brown (1976) points out that the many change events almost inevitably associated with divorce total "an ominous 258 [points]" on the stress scale developed by Holmes and Rahe (1967) and notes that "80 % of those who scored above 300 on this scale became pathologically depressed, had heart attacks, and developed other ailments" (p. 407). Brown considers the reduction of the attendant stress to be a primary objective of divorce counseling.

Treatment in this first phase was essentially crisis intervention, and the active techniques typical of this approach were utilized. Mr. Toman was encouraged to ventilate the turbulent feelings he was experiencing, and the helper, in addition to serving as an strongly empathic listener, offered explanatory comments that placed many of these reactions within the understandable framework of crisis. In order to increase Mr. Toman's knowledge of the normalcy of much of his turmoil, he was supplied with reading material on common fears and attitudes toward divorce. Finally, some simple relaxation exercises were practiced in the treatment session and utilized by Mr. Toman as a means of reducing some of the stress he was experiencing and consequently giving him a tangible method of coping with his fear of a further heart attack.

Accepting major life change. As the crisis subsided, Mr. Toman became more comfortable in facing the fact that within a few months his life was to undergo a major change. Although he was no longer acutely uncomfortable, he still had many questions about how he would be able to cope with the divorce and his unwilling return to a single life. He and the clinician agreed to work together for another two or three months with the goal of preparing him for this transition. In a certain sense he was already alone even though he and his wife were still living in the same house. Despite this nominal proximity they followed entirely different schedules, occupied separate bedrooms, seldom had a meal together, and talked only when absolutely necessary.

The major theme of therapy during this phase was one of accepting and coping with the major life change that was about to be thrust upon him. As this focus was more specifically examined, some of its goals became extremely practical. For example, how could Mr. Toman increase his ability to take care of his own needs in anticipation of the time when he would be living alone? In tasks related to this he began to wash his own laundry, shop for groceries, and cook more of his meals at home. Similarly, almost all of his social life for more than twenty years had revolved around his role as father, husband, and family member. Again, discussion and task assignments centered on identifying interests and activities that he could develop and actively locating new friends and social contexts where he could share these interests. Finally, although he was convinced that because of his religious convictions he himself could take no initiative in seeking divorce, Mr. Toman began to reflect on some of the ways in which his personal values would be challenged. At the urging of the therapist, he arranged an interview with his clergyman to discuss his religious status and to seek out information on his church's current views on such questions as sexuality and remarriage.

Dealing with impending separation. As work concluded on the previous phase and Mr. Toman saw himself as at least moderately ready to reenter the single life, it became apparent that his wife was about to initiate divorce proceedings. In one of their rare conversations she told him that she had consulted an attorney and expected that a divorce petition would be filed within a few weeks. Despite having anticipated the divorce for some time, Mr. Toman felt a renewed surge of the anger and anxiety that had troubled him at the very beginning of treatment. It became necessary to reapply, in milder form, the crisis intervention procedures that had characterized this first phase. Thus Mr. Toman was again supported in openly expressing his aroused emotions, and the therapist encouraged him to resume the relaxation exercises that had been helpful earlier.

By this point it was apparent that treatment was no longer explicitly short term and that contact with Mr. Toman would most likely continue for some time. However, the therapist deliberately kept the intervention goal-oriented, in the conviction that this not only would provide an effective form of service but also would avoid encouraging undue dependency on Mr. Toman's part. A new contract was negotiated, aimed at supporting Mr. Toman through the physical separation from his wife. Three main goals were important to him: (1) coping with his renewed anger and stress, (2) working on the altered relationship with his children that would be necessary as divorce became a reality, (3) helping him to deal with certain of the concrete aspects of negotiating a divorce settlement and moving to new living quarters.

Perhaps the simplest aspect of this phase was that of reducing Mr. Toman's renewed stress to manageable proportions. The other areas of concern progressed more slowly, and in major respects the therapeutic stance during this phase was markedly different. That is to say, the earlier phases of counseling had involved a rather behavioral orientation in which general concerns were translated into concrete objectives and related tasks. In contrast, in these sessions many of Mr. Toman's tangible worries—"What can I tell the children about the divorce?" "Should I accept my wife's ideas about dividing the property?"—were discussed in relation to such major themes as personal integrity, aspirations, and values and the feelings of competency and self-worth these engendered. The helping strategy thus became one of examining the specific questions confronting Mr. Toman as aspects of broader psychological and emotional issues—a process, of course, much more reminiscent of psychodynamically oriented therapy than the behavioral methods previously employed. This shift in emphasis was influenced by the clinician's perception that at this point Mr. Toman was not in need of specific direction in his life, but was attempting to place particular elements of the ongoing experience of separation and divorce into a comprehensible framework of value and belief.

Reacting to life alone. The final segment of counseling with Mr. Toman took place over a two-month period following the physical separation of the couple. Mr. Toman had moved into his own apartment but almost immediately began to find himself lonely and depressed. Two major goals were negotiated for this concluding phase of therapy: (1) to continue the build-up of social interests and new friendships he had begun much earlier, and (2) to start looking at himself as a single person and, particularly, considering what this meant to him in terms of relationships with women.

The focus on expanding his social activities was handled through a combination of reflective discussion of his needs and periodic task assignments directed at an identified area of interest. Some of this reflection and activity was no different than that engaged in by all persons attempting to expand their social and recreational network, but other aspects were peculiarly related to the divorce experience. Emily Brown (1976), in her highly informative discussion of divorce counseling, speaks of the "rapid and massive change which is triggered by the physical separation" (p. 400) and reviews research findings which identify this juncture as the point of greatest trauma. For Mr. Toman the physical transition provoked two central emotional issues: he worried about the possibility of mounting loneliness and isolation if he were unable to continue his efforts to seek new affiliations, and, perhaps even more strongly, he feared that in any intimate relationship his sexual functioning (long abandoned with his wife) would fail. The major goals of this final phase tended to be interrelated. Considering his role as a single person, for example, faced Mr. Toman with attitudinal and value issues related to intimacy, sexuality, and so on that in turn played an essential part in how he would choose to develop new relationships. Once again the task assignments served to firmly direct him to the interpersonal milieu where these choices had to be made.

A follow-up interview four months later found Mr. Toman functioning reasonably well. His overall adjustment was good and his social life relatively active. He found himself experiencing occasional episodes of loneliness or boredom, but he was generally optimistic about his ability to cope with his new life. He had begun some very tentative dating, but his apprehension that he would be unable to achieve satisfactory sexual functioning in a new relationship was still untested. He contacted the therapist a year after this follow-up session and was seen for two interviews. By this time he had moved into a close relationship with a middle-aged widow and was seriously contemplating remarriage. His description of this budding relationship was highly positive, and, contrary to his fears, its sexual aspects were very rewarding to him. As his essential dilemma was around the conflict between his religious beliefs and the question of remarriage, he was referred to a religious counselor to pursue these issues.

SOME FINAL CONSIDERATIONS

It will be apparent that many of the same principles, techniques, and strategies that govern regular brief treatment are also employed in what I have called goal-oriented extended treatment. The major difference, of course, lies in the lengthier period of contact between therapist and client. Yet even within this larger span of time, goals are specified for each distinct segment of treatment and care is exercised to stipulate reassessment points that are sufficiently close that both client and clinician remain aware of the approaching evaluation. It would be highly detrimental to this process if the time limits of a given segment were ignored and treatment allowed to assume an entirely open-ended character. Thus in many respects adherence to time constraints is even more important in this type of extended treatment. Further, as in the briefer time-limited variants, it is the helper who must assume the major responsibility to maintain this central aspect of the treatment structure.

The description of goal-oriented extended treatment and the examples of brief intervention given earlier in this chapter can be viewed as representative of the process of short-term therapy but are by no means intended to exhaust its complexities or possibilities. Other illustrations will be offered in succeeding chapters, and I will return to some of the examples given in this chapter to illustrate certain specific details of the interventive process. Before concluding this expository examination of brief (or goal-oriented) treatment, however, several general features require attention.

For instance, evident throughout the illustration of goal-oriented extended treatment—and perhaps even more apparent in the briefer variations described earlier—is the influence of what Kanfer (1979) has called the *instigative* approach to therapy:

> This strategy presumes that behavior change occurs *between* therapy sessions and that the "talk sessions" serve mainly to explore objectives, train the client in methods, and motivate him to modify his extra-therapeutic environment and to apply learning principles to his own behavior. In this sense the patient learns to become his own therapist. During sessions, assigned tasks are practiced, tactics are discussed, and a favorable orientation toward change is created [p. 189].

Kanfer contends that an instigative approach can avoid many of the difficulties with generalization that have plagued therapeutic practice. That is to say, all therapies have wrestled with the problem of ensuring that the changes that may take place within the therapeutic session are paralleled by similar changes in the client's daily life. Practically speaking, it has simply been assumed that if the client becomes more open and self-disclosing, let us say, within the therapeutic relationship, then identical movement is taking place in other relationships. The instigative strategy of viewing the therapy sessions as secondary to a primary emphasis on planned changes outside the session is a deliberate attempt to bypass the generalization dilemma by focusing directly upon the client's natural world.

Similarly running through all the variants of time-limited treatment that I have described is an underlying *educational* stance that, in many respects, is in opposition to the more prevalent philosophies of therapeutic helping. Quite aside from whether one subscribes to a disease model for explaining the development of emotional and social disturbance, most clinicians (whether psychodynamic, behavioral, or humanistic in theoretical orientation) have continued to utilize a medical model of practice. From this viewpoint the client is seen as a sufferer whose difficulties need to be individually diagnosed and treated by a professionally trained practitioner. Instead of necessarily following the medical paradigm of study, diagnosis, and treatment, the practitioner influenced by the educational model tends to see the therapeutic endeavor as fundamentally concerned with the *teaching* of the essential knowledge and interpersonal skills needed for effective living. Thus the practitioner is primarily a provider of important information and skills to individuals, troubled or otherwise, who might wish to employ these learnings in better managing their lives. Guerney (1977) has extensively discussed this perspective on helping:

> Viewing matters in this light, essentially as matters for educational effort, it seems far less important for the helper to discover what is wrong in a relationship, or why it went wrong, than to provide clients with appropriate knowledge, training and experience aimed at the future—that is, aimed at overcoming the difficulties or accomplishing the relationship goals in question. Usually, once one knows what clients wish to accomplish, not much time needs to be spent in finding out what makes them behave the way they do (diagnosis) and still less in finding out how they got the way they are (genesis). Rather, it is assumed that by far the most expeditious approach is immediately to begin: (1) teaching them what it is they need to know (providing the rationale); (2) establishing the appropriate life experience they need to elicit such behavior (providing practice); (3) helping them perfect their skills (providing supervision); and (4) increasing the use of skills in appropriate everyday situations (fostering generalization) [p. 20].

Although it shares some common ground with the instigative approach discussed earlier, the educational model of clinical practice carries other implications. It approaches the client as an individual in need of information or skill, as a student willing to learn, rather than as a patient who must be healed. The role of the helper is one of identifying the pertinent learnings that might be offered and, in conjunction with the client, deciding if these are suitable to the goals that the client wishes to achieve. As Guerney points out, such a stance reduces the need for a finely tuned diagnostic assessment and instead suggests that helpers must be able to clearly explain the benefits and limitations of their expertise so that the client can make a knowledgeable choice.

Finally, despite the obvious employment of a number of interventive strategies drawn from behavioral and social learning theory, it should be apparent that many of the techniques characteristic of the psychodynamic approaches can also be incorporated into brief intervention. In the work with Mr. Toman, for example, there were several points where major life themes were examined in a reflective and clarifying manner in order to enable him to thoughtfully consolidate his troubled value and belief system. Similarly, there were points with Mr. Jurecko where his attitudes toward himself and his work situation were carefully explored as a means of enhancing his awareness of their relationship to his anger outbursts.

Although later chapters will examine interventions such as behavior rehearsal and social skill training, techniques commonly considered behavioral, I think it is important to emphasize that this choice is entirely pragmatic rather than ideological. That is to say, any strategy for change must be evaluated in relation to the data supporting its usefulness in practice. Behavioral techniques have established a level of effectiveness that cannot be disregarded and additionally are often highly relevant to the limited and specific goals of short-term intervention. Yet at the same time there is at least broad substantiation for the effectiveness of psychodynamically influenced therapy. The study by Sloane and his colleagues (1975), for example, clearly establishes that short-term psychodynamic therapy benefits its recipients. Beyond the immediate question of outcome validation, there is no doubt that such techniques as reflection, clarification, and, in general, the attempt to insightfully examine important attitudinal and value themes must play a part in the repertoire of clinicians of all theoretical persuasions.

The issue becomes one of integrating a variety of strategies for inducing personal and behavioral change into a meaningful practice repertoire. This does not mean that one has to use all the techniques all the time, in some sort of "democratic" melange, but it definitely suggests that practice should not be confined within a narrow technical and theoretical range. The problem is one of selectivity. Perhaps the particular phase with Mr. Toman where reflective and clarifying techniques became predominant will illustrate this point. It will be remembered that this represented a stage in the contact where he was less concerned with what to do than with his need to understand the impinging effect of an unwanted event—the impending divorce—upon his existing value system. At this time, therefore, the therapeutic need was not for action but for reflection, and techniques pertinent to this latter goal became highly salient.

The synthesis required by a pluralistic approach, then, does not require that one regard the various theories and techniques as equivalent or interchangeable, but that the practitioner develop an appreciation of the differing purposes and goals that may be served by each approach or strategy. This allows for a knowledgeable and sensitive matching of client need and appropriate clinical knowledge and skill. An overriding concern, however, is that the clinician possess a sufficiently comprehensive range of interventive knowledge and skill that such selectivity is possible.

Chapter 4

The Initial Interview: Basic Goals

If therapy is to end properly, it must begin properly—by negotiating a solvable problem and discovering the social situation that makes the problem necessary.

—Jay Haley, 1976

First impressions can be confusing and inaccurate, yet they can also be of immense importance in establishing the tone and character of a human encounter. The initial interview in clinical practice, a matter of one hour, perhaps less, can significantly shape the outcome of whatever counseling may follow. Indeed, for many clients the helping experience begins and ends at this point, as they are screened out by the therapist or, more often, screen themselves out. Like political refugees, unwilling to endure or accept the restrictions they perceive will be placed upon their freedom, clients will exercise their option to "vote with their feet." It is therefore worthwhile to spend some time examining the initial interview in order to understand the essential elements needed at this vital entry point into short-term treatment. Chapter 5 will discuss the actual process and management of the first session.

Many private practitioners seem to have a finely tuned appreciation for the nuances of the initial interview. This is not necessarily due to the greater skill of the private practitioner as compared with the agency-based worker, but may be a function of an economic variable. The private practitioner's livelihood is dependent upon a refined ability to engage clients in an ongoing and workable relationship. The agency worker, on the other hand, can always turn to the agency's intake pool or waiting list for another case if a client drops out of treatment. Private practitioners, with the exception of a relatively few well-established individuals, do not have this luxury. Therefore, their skills in managing the initial engagement process—"hooking" the client— become quite polished.

Time limitations are present from the first moment of contact with the client; the therapist has about fifty minutes—sometimes less—to establish a relationship that can make helping possible. Within these time constraints a number of events must occur in the interchange between helper and client that will positively influence the projected venture of therapy. Thus, although the initial interview is inextricably bound to whatever may transpire in the future, it can be seen as having a reality of its own, as complete in itself and generating its own compelling demands. From this perspective it is surprising that this aspect of clinical practice has been so little examined and is so often regarded as simply a prelude to the more serious business that will follow.

The individual needing help, caught up in any of a range of troubling emotions or struggling and distracted by some problematic life situation, is hardly in a position to contribute greatly to the success of the first meeting. Clients are usually upset and distressed by their difficulties, infected with hopelessness about achieving any solution, sometimes reluctant to reveal the extent of their misery, and, as often as not, distrustful, even suspicious of the therapist.

The responsibility to create an atmosphere where learning, problem solving, or change can take place falls squarely upon the therapist. The initial interview therefore cannot be a random encounter, a social conversation, an inquiry into pathology, an exercise in "labeling," or a veiled interrogation in which the client must establish his or her "suitability" for service. Rather, it should be a process of negotiation, aimed at discovering a mutually agreeable purpose for counseling, yet a process firmly guided by the professional competence and values of the helper.

This suggests quite strongly that the therapist should be active and direct in the initial interview and at the same time should maintain a careful respect for the perspective offered by the client. In most instances of short-term helping the life problem of greatest concern to the client will become the goal of helping: parents who have difficulty in disciplining their children should learn how to discipline; married couples who can't talk together need to develop meaningful ways of communicating; the individual who is depressed about finding work needs assistance in obtaining employment, and so on. These and many others are all legitimate and important problems that can profoundly affect the life of the client and those around him.

The brief therapist not only should be willing to grapple seriously with such common difficulties, but should have a wide-ranging knowledge of problem-solving and change methods pertinent to their resolution. Additionally and perhaps most importantly, the effective helper has a highly developed ability to influence people to utilize such change methods toward the attainment of their chosen life goals. Skillful management of the initial interview is a critical first step in this process.

As the first interview begins, the therapist must realize that, given the client's emotional distress, lack of skill in coping with problems, or fearfulness in facing intense personal difficulty, the likelihood of a successful beginning is low. Unless the helper, in a planned way, initiates activity directed toward several vital and basic goals, it is quite possible that this human encounter, like others the client has experienced, will end in failure and disappointment. This chapter will discuss in some detail five essential goals of the initial interview:

1. Creating a hopeful atmosphere
2. Demonstrating explicit understanding of the client's emotional state

3. Locating one or two major problems in living
4. Establishing a contract to work upon a designated problem
5. Setting a time limit for service and giving the client an initial task

I will examine the theoretical rationale for each of these goals and their relationship to each other and to the overall purposes of the initial interview. It will be apparent that there are a number of ways of accomplishing each goal, depending upon the style and personal characteristics of the therapist, but each goal must be realized at least in part if the initial interview is to accomplish its major purpose—providing a sound beginning for effective helping.

It should be noted that throughout this and the next chapter my assumption will be that the therapist who conducts the first session will also be the ongoing helper. Fortunately, the once prevalent practice of an "intake interview" conducted by a separate practitioner is becoming a relic of the past. The minority of agencies that still retain this anachronistic practice should realize that, despite some minor organizational convenience, it can seriously increase drop-out and premature termination rates.

Creating Hope

We should not be surprised to find that the client's sense of hope—in technical terms, motivation—is at a very low ebb as he or she enters the initial interview. The client would not be a client—a person in need of help—if his or her own reserves of hope were not drained. It falls upon the therapist, then, to contribute a different viewpoint in which the possibility of change is implicit and in which hope, at some level, can begin to emerge. This is not to say that the helper should be naively or blindly reassuring, but it does emphasize that some modicum of hope is essential. Unless this first encounter between client and therapist does something to enhance the client's belief that his or her situation can possibly be different—to give some flicker of hope, however slight—then the chances of successful helping are considerably diminished. As Harry Stack Sullivan (1954) has stressed, the client expects and must receive some benefit from the interview. Gaining a sense of hope is a particularly important kind of benefit, and although the helper often has to work on this facet of the therapeutic process with considerable delicacy, there is no goal in the initial interview with greater consequence.

To a great extent the creation of hope, and the resulting enhancement of the client's willingness (and ability) to cope, flows from intangible aspects of the counselor's own belief system and the manner in which these beliefs are conveyed to the troubled individual. If the therapist is pessimistic about life or perfectionistic in attitude, or subscribes to theoretical frameworks which disparage the human potentiality for change, then little of a hopeful nature will be conveyed to the client. On the other hand, if the therapist has a personal outlook that is optimistic, a well-developed tolerance for human frailty, and theoretical beliefs that are supportive of these views, then the intangible aspects of hope are much more likely to be conveyed.

The question, then, is how hope can best be given within the context of the initial interview. As we are all aware, the conventional social response to the dejected person is reassurance—in effect, a direct attempt to counter the sufferer's prevailing belief system with new beliefs intended to restore hope. In its common-sense versions such reassurance is often given in massive doses, accelerating in quantity and tempo if the recipient proves unresponsive. From a theoretical perspective, reassurance is essentially a cognitive intervention—an attempt to provide information and to change belief—and as far as it goes, it does have some merit. However, in the hands of the overconcerned friend or a clumsy professional it is all too frequently aimed at the least problematic aspect of the sufferer's belief system and consequently has little effect.

Social learning theory offers an important insight into this issue. Bandura (1977a, 1977b) identifies two major sets of beliefs governing human activity. In contemplating a particular decision or action or in the process of carrying out a series of steps toward a chosen goal, we must make two judgments almost simultaneously. We must decide what behaviors, broadly speaking, are likely to achieve the desired result, and we must estimate our ability to carry out these behaviors. The first of these cognitive events Bandura calls "outcome expectations," while the second he refers to as "efficacy expectations." He reviews a number of research studies which suggest that the inhibition of action or the arousal of incapacitating emotions is more likely to be related to efficacy expectations—the judgment of personal capability—than to issues of outcome. From this viewpoint it is the weakened or inappropriate efficacy beliefs of the troubled person that are most potent in arousing negative affect—anxiety, tension, fear, and consequently hopelessness—which, in turn, inhibits the ability to act.

Similar views have been advanced from other theoretical perspectives. For example, Jerome Frank's (1961, 1978) work on the concept of "mastery" and his discussion of the weakened morale characteristic of psychiatric patients and Robert White's (1963) postulation of "effectance" and "competance" as independent ego energies concerned with "adaptation and with the governing of behavior by reality" (p. 24) both identify a like theme.

It is unfortunate, then, that reassurance, as it is commonly given, aims at imparting information of an optimistic and positive nature about outcome rather than efficacy. The crisis victim is assured that life is not as painful as it appears or that it will sooner or later improve; the anxiety-ridden individual is told that his fears are unfounded. These troubled people may be offered advice for the practical solution of their difficulties that, to the chagrin of the giver, they seem patently incapable of grasping.

None of this, of course, taps the powerful current of shattered morale, the pervasive belief that one is incapable of acting or, even more ominously, bound to fail. In instances where social reassurance is directed toward the troubled person's debased sense of efficacy, little is typically offered except injunctions to "buck up" or "get a grip on yourself," identifying a critical problem but providing only an ineffectual—even exasperated— directive toward resolution.

This discussion underscores the therapist's responsibility to attempt deliberately to instill hopefulness in whatever manner is pertinent and responsive to the client's struggle. At a minimum the therapist's actions—in the spirit of the Hippocratic injunction "First do no harm"—should not contribute in any way to a decrease in the client's ability to cope. This can happen, however, if the therapist's activities, whether through incompetence or misdesign, significantly subtract from the client's morale.

While such issues as the therapist's theoretical beliefs and philosophical stance play an important role in enhancing the client's sense of hopefulness, there are also many minor operations—redefining, relabeling, explanation, persuasion, and suggestion are only a few examples—through which the helper can also augment hope. In these instances—and I will discuss such strategies more fully in the following chapter—a cumulative effect is intended. That is to say, through the repetition of such techniques a gradual building of a hopeful atmosphere will occur, or at least the downward slide into discouragement and resignation will be halted.

Demonstrating Understanding

Almost without exception, theoretical and clinical descriptions of the therapeutic process have emphasized the importance of the helper's ability to empathize with the client's feelings. In addition to this consensus within the clinical literature, a substantial body of empirical research (Truax and Carkhuff, 1967; Truax and Mitchell, 1971) has supported the position that empathic understanding (along with the accompanying facilitative qualities of respect and genuineness) is essential, though not sufficient, for successful helping. While later studies have modified this view

(Parloff et al., 1978), establishing an emotional bond continues to be a central element in the helping process.

During the initial interview and especially in its early moments, the helper's demonstration of an understanding of the client's emotional state is critical. It cannot be overemphasized, however, that this understanding must be explicitly demonstrated, as therapists (even those of considerable experience) often mistake a sympathetic listening posture or an intellectual grasp of the client's emotions as representing accurate empathic response. Careful study of the definitions and examples of accurate empathic understanding offered by Carkhuff (1969) or Hammond et al. (1977) should be helpful in dispelling this notion.

Accurate empathy means that the therapist not only identifies the major emotion (or emotions) the client is expressing but clearly includes these in his response to the client. Thus if the client is expressing considerable dissatisfaction and frustration about his job, then the therapist's response might be as simple as "Your job is really bothering you, really getting you down." If the client, through words or nonverbal cues, is clearly expressing sadness or anger, then this emotion must be openly and specifically recognized by the helper. This may sound obvious, yet it is amazing—even disconcerting—to observe how often helpers do not respond in this simple manner, but instead become caught up in such peripheral matters as information gathering or diagnostic evaluation. A short verbatim passage from an initial interview with a troubled young woman will further illustrate the therapist's efforts to establish emotional connection through response to feeling:

Client: I don't know where to start really, It's just my whole life is such a mess right now. I just really don't know where to start. It's everything. (Sighs)

Therapist: It's like a lousy, lousy feeling about yourself.

Client: My job's a mess and I just—it's just everything. I don't— you know, I go to work but I just don't think I'm really catching on to what I'm supposed to be catching on to at work. I've been working there for six months but I just don't feel I'm learning what I should have learned. I still feel that I don't know what's going on and I just—

Therapist: (Interrupts) Am I following you? You're uncertain whether you're managing at work, keeping up with the job.

Client: I just—I don't know if I can do the job. I don't know if I can learn it.

Therapist: You're really doubtful, really uncertain.

In this brief excerpt, occurring at the very beginning of the initial interview, the helper's almost exclusive effort is to establish emotional contact with the client through response to feeling. All matters of content are secondary to this goal. Where the client works, the nature of her job, her age and education, whether she lives alone or with her family, what events in her life have led her to her present dilemma, and any of a multitude of other facts do not matter at this point. The therapist concentrates on the emotional dimension—the person in pain—and consistently directs his attention and response to this facet of the client's experience.

The client and helper are engaged in a truly human dialogue with the helper taking an active role in understanding the problematic emotions the client is undergoing about herself and her immediate world. At first the therapist can make only a general response to the client's global statement of turmoil, but even this general response is framed in words that attempt to capture the personal struggle of the client—"It's like a lousy, lousy feeling about yourself." As the client becomes a little more specific about where the struggle is occurring, the helper does not hesitate to interrupt her in order to convey his understanding and maintain his participation in the dialogue. When his identification of a particular feeling proves too mild, the therapist intensifies his response—"really doubtful, really uncertain"—as the exchange continues.

Accurate empathic understanding, carried out in this simple yet powerful manner, serves several purposes. There is no doubt that people respond to a person whom they perceive as understanding of their feelings. That is to say, they become more trusting of such a person, talk more about themselves, and in general are more likely to continue contact. Thus Truax and Mitchell (1971) found in their review of research studies that clients will tend to increase their self-exploration—their revealing of self—in response to highly empathic counselors.

Examining the issue of continuance in treatment, Waxenberg (1973) found that families were more likely to continue past the initial interview when they were offered high levels of accurate empathy in the first meeting. Waxenberg's findings are of particular interest because she found that nonwhite (black and Chicano) families were as likely as white families to remain in treatment, regardless of the ethnicity of the therapist, if the level of accurate empathy in the initial interview was sufficiently high.

In the light of the very high drop-out rates often seen in minority populations, this is a critical finding. In effect, immediate and accurate response to feeling in the early stages of the initial interview not only forms an emotional bridge between client and helper but plays a significant role in encouraging the client's return. Conversely, it is apparent that the therapist who neglects emotional response and emphasizes, for example, diagnostic exploration may formulate many brilliant diagnostic statements but will find that relatively few clients continue in treatment. This sort of practitioner is a familiar figure in many agencies—full of elaborate explanations about clients who were "not ready," "too sick," or whatever is the currently fashionable pathological label. It is all too easy, in the peculiar confabulations of the mental health professions, to blame the victim for the deficiencies of the perpetrator.

Furthermore, the need for empathic understanding may be especially acute in the person in crisis, the very sort of individual whose emotional disruption has provoked a request for help. Direct and accurate response to the feelings that are affecting such a person not only offers understanding but can foster hope. For instance, discovery by a troubled young woman such as the one in the preceding dialogue, that another human being is able to face her most frightening, disheartening, or angry feelings squarely can significantly influence her perception of her situation. This does not mean that the distressing emotions change, but the client is now able to see herself as less alone, less alienated from the world. Grier and Cobbs (1968) have poignantly captured this facet of the helping encounter:

> The essential ingredient is the capacity of the therapist to love his patient—to say to him that here is a second chance to organize his inner life, to say that you have a listener and companion who wants you to make it [p. 180].

Thus the helper's demonstration of accurate empathic understanding not only plays a vital role in establishing a human relationship between therapist and client but interacts with the equally critical goal of establishing hope. It should be emphasized, however, that I am advocating the use of empathic response, not in the Rogerian sense of a total technique, but rather within the context of a variety of other, direct or indirect therapeutic tactics.

It may be belaboring the obvious to point out that the problems people bring to therapy contain important feeling dimensions which are interacting with their behaviors and beliefs. Indeed, for the person in crisis, it is the very existence of strong and painful affect that is the core of the problem, and not necessarily the content of her or his immediate life situation. In order to assess the problems the client wishes to solve and devise a workable plan of intervention, it may be necessary to determine the specific emotions involved. There are differences, for example, between the individual who feels frustrated by a given problem and one who responds to the same problem with sadness or anxiety. Such differences may not only identify a style of response to life but suggest the choice of helping strategies. Thus the empathic responses of the helper will gently probe what is often a bewildering mass of emotion, identifying specific feelings and their connection to life events, and bit by bit will encourage the client's capacity to face them.

Finally, the therapist in short-term treatment is particularly concerned with assuming a position of influence in the life of the client. Without such influence the effects of the various strategies and techniques employed in time-limited treatment will be diluted and therefore less persuasive. This deliberate assumption of a position of influence is temporary and directed only toward the change goals that client and therapist negotiate, but it is essential for effective helping. People are much more likely to be influenced by someone who they believe understand them. As painful and unwanted feelings tend to predominate at times when people need therapeutic help, this dimension of their life must be explicitly understood. Empathic response builds both a human, intimate relationship and a considerable power. The therapist should recognize and respect not only the intimacy that is established but also the power that this can convey. Both are needed; neither can stand alone.

Identifying Problems in Living

Short-term treatment, as the previous chapters outlined, is aimed at helping people make the immediate changes in their lives that will reduce emotional distress, improve their relationships with significant others, solve difficult personal problems, and, by so doing, enhance their capacity for more satisfying living. All of these very general goals must be reduced to the specific difficulties, the problems in living, that a particular client is experiencing as help is requested.

In this formulation the client is seen as experiencing an undesirable emotional state in relation to a specific aspect of his or her current life. As Wood (1978) emphasizes, "The problem in living with which the client is struggling must be stated in clear and straightforward terms, preferably in plain English" (p. 451). This statement of the problem is developed as much as possible from the client's own description, although sometimes the therapist will have to guide and assist the process. The following examples, drawn directly from practice, are typical problem formulations:

- Mrs. A., a single parent, felt angry and frustrated about her inability to control the behavior of her adolescent son.

- A young man was depressed and anxious about his lack of confidence in relationships with women.
- A middle-aged couple, Mr. And Mrs. M., were extremely upset by the problems the husband was experiencing with sexual arousal.
- Mr. P. was suffering marked physical and emotional tension in the everyday course of his busy life.

Each of these brief examples could of course be much more explicitly defined, but they illustrate, however roughly, the kind of preliminary problem formulation that client and therapist will cooperatively develop in the initial interview. Wood summarizes the benefits of such direct problem formulation:

> Working with the client toward a simple and clear statement of the problem with which he or she wants help achieves two purposes: It helps the client begin to comprehend what he or she needs and wants to change in his or her life situation and what he or she wants to work toward; and it helps the worker achieve clarity and focus about the purpose of the interaction with the client or client system [1978, p. 451].

Reid and Epstein (1972) present a useful series of categories for conceptualizing the problems in living—in their terminology "target problems"—which may confront an individual. These will be briefly summarized:

1. *Interpersonal conflict.* A difficulty or conflict occurring in the relationship between two (or more) individuals, with particular reference to a situation in which neither feels free to withdraw from the relationship. This problem in living is of course most commonly seen in families, between husband and wife or parents and children, but can also occur in teacher-pupil, boss-worker, and other such relationships.

2. *Dissatisfactions with social relations.* This refers to situations where an individual client feels distressed about his or her relationships with others, although these significant others may not see the relationship as unsatisfactory, nor will there necessarily be conflict. Thus the client may picture his or her behavior as

unassertive or overly dependent or, in more general terms, may feel lonely and distant from others.

3. *Difficulties in role performance*. The client perceives a gap between his or her actual performance of an important role and the manner in which he or she would like to act. For example, a mother may see herself as too demanding of her children, or a student may not be able to involve herself in study.

4. *Reactive emotional distress*. This category is employed where the client's major concern is with the pronounced negative feelings that he or she is currently experiencing in life, rather than with the situation that provoked them. The situation itself may be in the past and therefore unchangeable, or it may be beyond the client's effective control.

5. *Problems of social transition*. In this category the individual is experiencing difficulty in moving from one social position, role, or situation to another. Examples include discharge from hospital, becoming a parent, getting a divorce, moving to a new city. Dislocation and abrupt, often unwanted change are the common theme, and the client is frequently bewildered and anxious about how to cope.

6. *Problems with formal organizations*. A type of conflict between the client and an antagonist that is an organization rather than person. Like interpersonal conflict, this is a situation where the client cannot simply ignore the other, but a relationship of some meaningful dimension must continue.

7. *Inadequate resources*. In these instances the client lacks specific and tangible resources such as money, food, employment, social activities, and so on. Selecting this category of problem in living as the focus of intervention implies that the client and helper are going to work together in a systematic way to attain the needed resources.

These categories are helpful in directing the helper toward the major areas of personal, interpersonal, or social dysfunction which may be affecting the client's current life. Although not inclusive, they are sufficiently comprehensive to subsume the majority of client requests under one or another category. Their most useful function, however, is not as a quasi-diagnostic device—the emphasis is not on pigeonholing a problem within a given category—but as a sort of systematized reminder to the helper that human difficulties are identifiable and concrete clusters of events occurring in the daily lives of clients. The *problem,* then, is not that an individual ''lacks ego strength'' or ''needs to develop explicit reinforcers,'' but that some meaningful aspect of life has become disrupted: a married couple quarrel frequently or can't enjoy sex; parents are overwhelmed by their parental responsibilities; an individual is overcome by the accumulation of everyday stress.

This is not to say that the therapist does not develop certain notions about the nature of the client's difficulties, based on a particular theoretical framework, or that he or she does not utilize this framework to formulate a possible interventive approach. Thoughtful activity of this sort is a very necessary part of the therapeutic role. There is no doubt that every therapist needs some way of organizing personal thoughts—especially in the peculiarly stressful and intense moments of the first session. As Norris Hansell (1973) has remarked, a theoretical framework can be remarkably comforting at such times. Such theoretical constructs, however, expecially in the highly goal-oriented context of brief therapy, are justifiable only if they are directly related to the process of problem resolution, and, in any case must never be confused with the actual problem.

None of this discussion should be taken as suggesting that there are not times when there may be a need to define or redefine the problem that the client presents in a way that makes it more workable or more specific. On the other hand, the helper should not regard the client's request as, by definition, superficial or irrelevant—such common mental health terms as ''presenting problem,'' ''complaint,'' or ''symptom'' all convey this demeaning notion. Reid and Epstein (1972) cogently warn against the dangers of ''double-agenda'' helping that this viewpoint can encourage—where the counselor apparently accepts the client's stated problem but implicitly decides that some other facet of the client's life is the "real" problem and bides his time until the client realizes this. Short-term treatment, in contrast, is usually a straightforward attempt to deal with the most immediately distressing life problem as this is directly negotiated and contracted with the client. A case illustration drawn from an article by Weinberger (1971) will illustrate this philosophy in action:

Mrs. B., a mother in her early twenties, felt both helpless and frustrated in coping with the temper tantrums of her four-year-old daugther. After an initial interview in which the specific dimensions of the difficulty were explored, the therapist initiated a six-session series of interviews. During the intervention Mrs. B. was, first, given information on the essential normalcy of her own and her child's reactions and, second, provided with instructions and encouragement in firmer handling of the troublesome behavior.

Many of the difficulties that helpers encounter at later stages of the interventive process can be seen as related to weaknesses in problem identification in the initial interview. The difficulties that were most meaningful to the client were identified only vaguely at this point, sometimes because the client was reluctant or mistrustful but as often as not because the helper became intrigued with peripheral concerns or simply didn't press for greater specificity.

Establishing a Contract

Toward the end of the initial interview, as the client's major problems in living become apparent, the therapist will initiate discussion about the possibility of an explicit agreement to work on one of these areas. This should be done in as simple and open a manner as possible.

Therapist: From what we've discussed I notice that you keep putting a lot of stress on how dissatisfied you are with your ability to make friends. Would you be willing to work with me on this difficulty?

Client: I don't know, it's so hard to say—sometimes I just don't think it's any use even trying. Do you think I could find out what keeps me from getting anywhere with people?

Therapist: I'm pretty certain that people can make some important changes in their lives, though sometimes it takes some real effort and you can feel awfully discouraged about trying it out. Are you interested in us working on this together?

Client: I guess so. (Pause) I don't know if it's any use, but I haven't got much to lose.

In this dialogue it should be noted how the therapist persistently and personally phrases the offer of counseling. There is an emphasis on "working with me" and on "us working together" which, in very plain language, suggests that the therapeutic process is a mutual endeavor of two concerned people. The therapist's choice of the verb "work" to characterize the helping process is also not accidental, but is a deliberate attempt to convey that activity on the part of both therapist and client will be expected. Beyond this, the concept of work as a valued and understandable human activity carries the implication that the process of change will be not mystical or exotic but simple and ordinary, perhaps even a little sweaty.

It is easy to overemphasize the impact of such phrasing or the choice of particular words. A therapist would be naive to believe that every careful distinction, every subtle nuance of tone or gesture, has an immediate and direct effect on the client. All too often clients are caught up in such stress that only the gross dimensions of the therapist's responses are readily apparent to them. Despite these reservations, I believe that attention must be paid to the therapist's words and nonverbal communication, as these, in their totality, contribute to an atmosphere, an ambience, that must be continued and accumulated with a careful persistence before its effects will prevail.

Similarly, the therapist cannot expect that the client will wholeheartedly grasp the offer of help. As the preceding fragment illustrates, the client's agreement may be tentative and clouded with discouragement and uncertainty. The essential point, however, is that the offer is clearly made and clearly accepted, no matter how weak the acceptance my be. If the client is not able to make even an ambivalent acceptance, then therapy, in its usual form, cannot proceed. At this juncture the therapist must fall back upon a secondary position, perhaps offering a further interview to consider the possibility of counseling. When the client's reluctance is obviously stronger—or if he or she plainly conveys disinterest—then the therapist may only be able to suggest that the client think about the notion of help and resume contact at some later time.

Setting a Time Limit and Giving a Task

After client and worker have reached an agreement, however tentative, to work together on a selected problem, two further steps remain that are especially important to initiating the process of planned short-term treatment. The first involves setting a time limit governing the duration of treatment; the second step entails assigning some activity to the client which can be carried out prior to the next therapy session. The time limit, of course, epitomizes the planned brevity of the helping process, while the task emphasizes the active, practical nature of change.

Short-term treatment, as earlier chapters have noted, comprises three or four sessions up to a maximum of fifteen interviews. As I have repeatedly emphasized, the time limit is explicitly conveyed to the client, most commonly at the end of the initial interview. The therapist takes on the responsibility to select a suitable time limit and to inform the client of this. Choosing a time limit is seldom an area of negotiation with the client but is formulated by the helper as a function of his professional judgment.

Certain issues concerning the selection and employment of time limits will be considered further in the next chapter. Three major points will be emphasized here:

First, there is no doubt that the explicit use of a time limit places pressures on helper and client alike and that these pressures affect both the scope and the pace of the helping process. Once a time limit has been defined—eight sessions, let us say— then the therapist realizes that she or he must strive to define the contracted problem in even more specific terms and, most critically, to choose and utilize a change strategy which will have definite impact. Most clients appear to be positively affected by the time limit, frequently finding the notion of a foreseeable end point encouraging and hopeful.

Second, it is often difficult for therapists to conceive of significant personal or emotional change taking place within a relatively limited period of time. Most therapists have been educated to place a higher value on lengthy and ambitious therapeutic ventures. Beginning helpers may have a sketchier notion of the therapeutic process yet may still share the bias common among the educated middle class that treatment should somehow be wide ranging and long lasting. Clients from lower-middle-class, working-class, or low socioeconomic backgrounds do not necessarily share this viewpoint, and indeed there have been times when I have found myself hard put to convince such a client that even three or four sessions did not constitute an unreasonably long period of treatment. In other words, it is well for therapists to keep in mind that belief in the primacy of lengthy therapeutic ventures—quite aside from empirical evidence challenging their effectiveness—is a predominantly middle-class bias that is not shared by large groups of potential clients.

Finally, although an explicit time limit is established at the beginning of treatment and the helper makes every effort to structure treatment within this time limitation, there is no doubt that a certain number of cases take longer. It is quite possible, in other words, to reach the predicted time limit and to see the desired goal still unattained. In such instances, therapist and client may negotiate a further series of sessions so as to continue the helping process toward its proper conclusions. The therapist, then, is well aware that the predicted time limit with any given client is not inviolable—more or less time may be required—but this should not be a temptation to omit or needlessly qualify the time limit in short-term treatment. If the helping process is to derive useful impact from the pressures of time, the time limit should be presented in a positive manner, neither hedged nor overemphasized, and the change strategies employed should be shaped so as to fit reasonably within the predicted number of sessions.

Homework tasks are frequently employed in brief therapy and serve at least two major functions. First, they help to emphasize the active nature of the process of change and to engage the client in the purposeful dimensions of this process. Second, the assignment of tasks, which characteristically are carried out between therapy sessions, symbolizes the need for change to take place in real life and thus tend to reduce client dependence on the therapist or the therapeutic setting. These important aspects of tasks, as well as many of the clinical subtleties that can enter into formulating or giving such directives to action, are discussed in detail in Chapter 7.

As the initial interview moves to its conclusion, the therapist is concerned to prescribe an assignment that will impart to the client that active participation will be expected. It is often difficult to devise a task at this point, for the therapist has only limited knowledge about the client and the salient aspects of the client's major life problems. These very difficulties, however, suggest the direction that the initial task can take. That is to say, the therapist will ask the client to carry out a task that will add such needed information—a task, in other words, that will further explore a selected aspect of the contracted problem.

For example, parents concerned about their child may be asked to keep daily notes on the circumstances in which the problem behaviors occur. A troubled marital couple can be asked to work out a written list of the areas in their relationship that each would like to see changed—or, more positively, the aspects of the relationship that each partner values. It is critical at this beginning point, not that the most pertinent and focused task be selected, but that the client's own participation be stimulated in a simple but direct manner.

It is often helpful to offer the client an explanation of the general purpose of the task. This too can be done in a straightforward manner, and indeed, it is best if the helper is as open and concrete as possible in any explanations that are given. For example, if one is instructing parents to record the behavior of their child as an initial task, the explanation might take the following form:

As we've talked here, it seems that the major difficulty we are going to have to work on is how to help Tommy make more friends and become more confident in how he gets along with other children. To get us started on this, I'd like to ask you to keep a daily record over the next week of every instance where you see him involved with another child. Keep a record of who he is with, what they do together, and anything else you might think is important. This will give us a much clearer idea, as we begin working together, of exactly how things go for Tommy in this area, what things he is managing all right, and exactly where he is having most difficulty.

The instructions would of course vary if the target problem involved aggressive behavior with other children or if the parents were concerned about their child's study habits. The essential focus would be similar, however, in that it would involve the attempt to define a very clear-cut task for the parents to undertake, a brief connection of this task to the problem-solving work that lies ahead, and the suggestion of an active approach to coping with difficulties.

Implicit in the use of tasks is the belief that change takes place most effectively and meaningfully where clients are encouraged to take an active role in their own lives. In comparison with the commonsense tactic of advice giving, the therapeutic utilization of tasks is very varied and subtle—although at the same time there is nothing shameful in admitting that there are definite commonalities. One difference lies in the manner in which the task is presented. Seldom if ever does the helper suggest that a particular task in itself is the solution to a problem. Rather, she or he explains that it represents a step along a pathway to resolution.

Similarly, tasks are conceptualized and presented as miniature learning experiences—offering opportunity for observation, experimentation, and challenge—and the therapist is careful to avoid presenting a task as involving anything so definitive as success or failure. The issue is not the outcome of a particular task, but the task's contribution, however small, to an ongoing process of change.

Chapter 5

The Initial Interview: Process

If the therapist fails to participate actively in the treatment, events will pass him by, ambiguity as to both process and goals will intervene, and what began as time-limited psychotherapy will become diffuse, indefinite, long-term psychotherapy.
　　　　　　　　　　　　　　　　　　　—James Mann, 1973

Clinical practitioners are beginning to pay more attention to the specific techniques that are needed to encourage clients to become involved participants in the therapeutic process. It has become clearer that the therapist, too, must play an active part in the engagement process, particularly in the initiation of short-term treatment. Rather than assume that motivation for help, for instance, is simply a factor to be assessed by the therapist as an aspect of the many other diagnostic functions of the initial interview, there is a growing recognition that, within realistic limits, there is much that the helper can do to increase client motivation.

In the preceding chapter I outlined and discussed a series of goals that the short-term therapist must strive to achieve in the initial interview. These included arousing hope, responding to the predominant emotions troubling the client, defining the immediate life problems that precipitated the request for help, negotiating a contract with the client to work on one or two of the most important of these difficulties, and, finally, defining a time limit and giving the client a task to carry out.

Accomplishing all this within an hour or so may seem like a

104

formidable task. Yet the experienced brief therapist can usually manage at least a reasonable approximation of each of these goals within the confines of a single interview. As in any learned skill, there is no doubt that simply gaining experience in working within a given framework adds to one's facility and confidence.

A major aid in attaining facility with first interviews is to develop a cognitive map—a structure in the mind—of the typical process of this vital session. Short-term treatment is highly dependent upon such heuristic schemas, and these occur and reoccur at many different levels during the interventive process. The better the clinician is able to visualize a systematic sequence for any aspect of the helping process, whether he is concerned with management of the initial contact, ways of quickly building an influential relationship, or implementation of interventive strategies, the more effectively will the self-imposed time constraints of brief therapy be utilized.

It is obvious that the use of schemas of this sort often involves a deliberate simplification of seemingly complex situations. The practitioner must be willing to accept the risk this entails with the conviction that more often that not the path of simplification achieves as good an outcome as more complex (and consequently lengthier) approaches. The consistent finding that with similar problem and client groupings brief treatment is generally as effective as a lengthier approach justifies such a stance.

Additionally, the helper practicing short-term therapy needs an expanded appreciation of the many ways in which the engagement process can be refined and shaped. It is not enough that the clinician be active—this activity must be purposefully related to achieving the basic goals of engagement. Outlining such a process, in relation to a series of rough stages, and attempting to give some illumination of the techniques that support each stage will be the task of this chapter.

It will also be apparent that the initial interview in short-term practice, as I briefly noted much earlier, is the first (and perhaps most significant) instance of the planned use of time. That is to say, the helper must be acutely aware, as the first session begins, that a number of tasks need to be accomplished within a limited period of time. This awareness should serve to place a constructive pressure upon the therapist to pace the interview around these goals rather than to permit the process to be governed by whatever intriguing "dynamics" may be apparent in the client or in the very process itself. The purpose of facilitating progress toward these goals should take precedence over anything except the most compelling concerns or happenings. Thus the helper must be exquisitely aware of the passage of time during the initial interview and, where needed, must control her or his own range of exploration in relation to this limitation. Similarly, the therapist will take the responsibility of placing controls upon client activity in order to accomplish the tasks of the initial interview in as economical a manner as possible.

This is not to say that the therapist, in order to manage the pertinent therapeutic tasks, will deliberately ignore the need of an extremely anguished client to talk about his or her pain. The goals and procedures of any therapeutic method must be cast aside in the face of a genuine emotional crisis of large proportions. However, what is more often the case in unplanned or unproductive initial interviews is that the client simply rambles on in a disorganized way, offering detailed descriptions of this or that problem, in the belief that this is what the helper wants to hear. The clinician, for lack of a better plan, either allows this to happen or, worse still, encourages it by supportive comments and interjections. The techniques and strategies discussed in the succeeding sections will offer the practitioner a viable alternative.

A Survey of Engagement Techniques

William Schwartz, in his foreword to Schulman's *The Skills of Helping* (1979), points out that there has been a marked reluctance on the part of the helping professions to identify specific therapeutic techniques and, in contrast, an almost inordinate emphasis on the more general principles of diagnosis and treatment. He succinctly poses the resulting dilemna:

> The neglect of means has produced a professional literature that is extremely thin in its description of practice. It is largely concerned with diagnosis, conceptual analysis, philosophy and abtract discussion [p. vii].

There is apparently a belief that clinicians must be encouraged to think in broad, inclusive terms and, along with this, a fear that to stress technique will lead to narrowness and rigidity in practice. I believe there is much to be said for a concentration on the minutiae of technique. Instead of fostering rigidity or narrowness, the careful development of a range of technical skills can expand the clinician's capacity for flexibility and diversity of approach. With such a objective in mind, this section will examine a number of specific techniques that the therapist can employ, as needed, within the engagement process that is being attempted in the first interview. These techniques derive from three sources:

(1) research studies of the process of therapeutic intervention;

(2) the published transcripts, audiotapes, and videotapes of experienced therapists; and

(3) direct practice experience.*

The techniques can be roughly categorized in three major groups:

(1) relationship or influence-building strategies,

(2) educational or informational strategies, and

(3) management or survival strategies.

I will briefly survey a number of engagement techniques under each of these headings and, in later sections of this chapter, illustrate their employment throughout the major phases of the first session.

---

*Certain aspects of this discussion will be based upon previous writing (Wells, 1980) in which I examined engagement techniques and strategies from the perspective of marital and family therapy. Although the demands of these modes of treatment are somewhat different from those of one-to-one intervention, many of the same considerations apply within the engagement process.

RELATIONSHIP OR INFLUENCE-BUILDING STRATEGIES

Brief therapy is particularly dependent on the ability of the therapist to quickly establish an atmosphere in which the client not only feels understood but has enough trust and confidence in the clinician that the interventive strategies to be employed at a later phase will have sufficient impact. In contrast to conventional clinical practice, the emphasis in short-term treatment is on the rapid development of a significant relationship within the areas of pressing concern to the client. Of the techniques deliberately employed to expedite movement toward this goal, five predominate:

Socializing. This is a technique employed during the first few moments of an initial interview where the therapist very briefly interacts with the client at a social level. It is used as a transition from the social level of the preliminary contact into the more serious therapeutic conversation that will follow. Some of the nuances of this seemingly innocuous engagement strategy will be discussed later in this chapter in the section on the inception phase of the first interview.

Facilitation. Almost every therapeutic approach emphasizes the empathic ability of the clinician, the ability to respond immediately and accurately to the emotional state of the client, whether such feelings are expressed directly or indirectly.

As the preceding chapter emphasized, empathic response should be seen as a very literal process in which the therapist (1) reflects back the emotions the client has openly expressed, (2) explicitly labels major feelings that are expressed through the client's nonverbal behavior, or (3) identifies important feelings that are simply a part of the human context of the problem situation being described, as, for example, sadness from a loss or frustration when thwarted. In most instances, the most common and ordinary terms are employed. Words such as ''worried,'' ''angry,'' ''sad,'' ''relieved,'' ''disappointed,'' ''happy,'' ''scared,'' and ''concerned,'' should permeate the dialogue between helper and client as the problem situation and its emotional repercussions are explored.

3   *Joining or accommodating.* In this important engagement technique the helper attempts to convey to the client that there are similarities or parallels at an intellectual, social, or emotional level between helper and client. Although most obviously useful in family interviewing (Minuchin, 1974), where the therapist is often confronted with the task of engaging a hostile or tightly defended family group, the use of joining techniques is highly applicable in one-to-one intervention. Joining may involve minor bits of self-disclosure from the therapist or the use of humor and words and phrases particularly attuned to the personal or cultural style of the client (Bandler and Grinder, 1976). The technique is intended to foster identification between therapist and client and to expedite the clinician's assumption of a meaningful (though temporary) role within the client's social network.

4   *Mimicking.* This refers to a number of *nonverbal* ways in which the practitioner indicates human similarities between himself and the client. The technique serves the same purposes as joining but differs in its employment of the nonverbal rather than the verbal level of interchange. Minuchin (1974) calls this "mimesis" and suggests that such nonverbal responses are a natural human reaction in a close relationship. He offers some typical therapeutic examples:

> Experienced therapists perform mimetic operations without even realizing it. Mr. Smith takes off his coat and lights a cigarette. The therapist, who asks him for a cigarette, is aware of performing this as a mimetic operation. But he is unaware of taking off his own coat. As he talks with Mr. Smith, he also scratches his own head in a puzzled, fumbling way, which robs him of authority and increases his kinship with the puzzled, fumbling patient [pp. 128–129].

5   *Redefining or relabeling.* At a number of critical points in the initial interview the clinician may need to restate a remark by the client in such a manner that the words employed are less stigmatizing or blaming or, on the other hand, more hopeful. The

therapist's restatement may also suggest that there are different attitudes, emotions, or motivations underlying the client's behavior. For example, a client's manifest anxiety about a problem might be characterized as a more laudable "concern" to do something about it or as an understandable indication of its importance in his or her life. In either case, the purpose of this technique is to reduce dysfunctional emotional arousal and to begin to induce hope and understanding through the cognitive change effected by the relabeling or redefinition.

EDUCATIONAL OR INFORMATIONAL STRATEGIES

During the initial interview information necessarily flows two ways—from client to therapist and from therapist to client. Yet perhaps too often the therapist ends up with a good deal of data about the potential client, while the client has gained only the most indirect information about the therapist or the process of therapeutic intervention. There is a tendency for inexperienced therapists to assume that their clients are quite familiar with the expectations and demands of the process. Consequently, the practitioner will neglect to teach these vital norms. Most helping professionals are middle class and expect that clients share their own attitudes and values toward therapy. However, if the client has only a hazy notion of what therapy will be like, it is quite possible that many behaviors that appear to reflect "resistance" or "poor motivation" are merely uninformed attempts to respond to a new (and often puzzling) experience. Jerome Frank (1978) suggests that premature termination of therapy may be related to this issue of disparate expectations:

> Those who work with therapists-in-training in a clinic setting share the impression that a major reason why patients drop out of treatment is that they do not know what is supposed to be going on or how it can help them. Because they are in awe of the therapist, they politely answer his questions and he thinks everything is going well; meanwhile the patients are wondering what it is all about, until suddenly they quit without warning [p. 22].

At the same time the therapist also needs information about the client, and certain of the techniques in this category offer a means of managing this aspect of the initial interview. The therapist's mastery of a series of techniques for gaining precise information about the client's current functioning and major areas of difficulty is, of course, essential to the rapid engagement process of short-term treatment. Four main techniques serve in facilitating these related purposes of information gathering and client education:

Structuring. The techniques that fall under this general heading refer to the ways in which the clinician directly or indirectly conveys information about the process of treatment. Structuring may describe to the client what the therapist believes to be the most useful approach: "The main thing we will be doing in counseling is trying to understand the parts of your life that are causing you most stress" or "I'll be helping you to learn some specific ways in which you can better stand up to people." Lennard and Bernstein's (1960) content analysis of therapeutic interviews found that experienced therapists devoted significant portions of their input in early interviews to such activity.

On the other hand, structuring may emphasize what the client *should not do* and in such instances becomes an explicit control device. In brief therapy this type of structuring is usually employed to place restraints on the exploration and description of content areas judged to be irrelevant to the immediate goals of the engagement process. Thus once a major problem has been identified, the clinician may limit discussion to an examination of only this area.

Tracking. In its most general sense this term refers to comments and responses from the clinician that serve to encourage the client in conveying needed information (Minuchin, 1974). Additionally, tracking responses help to shape this information into the more specific and focused form required for short-term treatment. The client may be able to express his or her difficulties only in a confused or vague manner and thus may need considerable assistance from the practitioner in order to arrive at workable treatment goals. Tracking techniques offer a means of accomplishing this important task.

At its simplest level tracking consists of nothing more or less than brief nods, attentive posture and gaze, or subvocal interjections such as "Mmm-hmm," which indicate the therapist's interest in whatever the client is describing. In short-term treatment, however, tracking often involves a more active participation on the part of the helper in order to expedite the identification and exploration of problem areas suitable for intervention. The therapist will then utilize such devices as close-ended questions, queries about "critical incidents," or the written formulation of target problems in order to encourage and direct this process. Some of these focused aspects of tracking will be apparent as the process of the initial interview is described in later sections of this chapter.

Summarizing. This technique can be seen as a heightened form of tracking and, as the term indicates, involves the therapist's attempts to pull together important aspects of the client's difficulties or to test out the accuracy of the therapist's understanding of these problems. Summaries should be employed frequently throughout the initial interview in order to help maintain a focus and additionally as a way of concretely demonstrating to the client the therapist's interest and effort to comprehend. An active use of summaries can have the very beneficial effect of changing the climate of the initial interview from that of a monologue by the client, supported by brief practitioner reinforcements ("Uh-huh," "Go on"), to an active dialogue between two concerned people.

Normalizing. Through the use of normalizing techniques the practitioner conveys to the prospective client that the difficulties he or she is experiencing, or the emotional reactions that are troublesome, are understandable human responses or, in other instances, are not uncharacteristic of the client's environmental situation or life stage. However, it is important to remember that normalizing should not become simple reassurance. The underlying message of the normalizing response is not "Don't worry, everyone experiences this," but rather "I'm not surprised (or shocked) that you have these problems."

It must be stressed, moreover, that normalizing is not simply a clever tactic through which the clinician talks away the client's difficulties. The helper must have sufficient experience with the human condition to know that most, if not all, of the problems people bring to professionals are simply heightened versions of the difficulties that any of us may encounter. This is the essence to Sullivan's (1953) one-genus postulate: "We are all much more simply human than otherwise, be we happy and successful, contented and detached, miserable and mentally disordered or whatever" (p. xviii).

MANAGEMENT OR SURVIVAL STRATEGIES

Quite aside from the techniques intended to establish a relationship or educate the client in the ways of the therapeutic encounter, there are a number of techniques which help the therapist to contend with the difficult moments that can arise in the beginning phase of any close human relationship. I commented on this issue in relation to family and marital therapy in an earlier work (Wells, 1980):

> Beginning therapists can slide, almost unwittingly, into major difficulties in an initial interview and often find themselves experiencing painful stress during (and after) a session. Overly idealistic therapists struggle with conflicts between the apparent polarities of "manipulation versus genuineness" or "spontaneity versus structure" and consequently have great difficulty in achieving a workable style. Many seasoned therapists, however, come to realize that the personal and emotional survival of the therapist is paramount—not at the expense of the family, to be sure but in order to be able to offer effective help. Thus, such therapists, bit by bit, gain skill in using a series of techniques that help in this essential task of avoiding difficulties or, at the least, not making a bad situation any worse [pp. 86–87].

The relationship and educational techniques suggested earlier should be seen as the predominant techniques of the initial interview. Yet the management techniques represent highly useful ways for the clinician to navigate the sometimes difficult waters of the engagement process and, to my knowledge, are seldom openly discussed in the literature. Judiciously employed in the service of the client, these strategies can help to avoid otherwise disastrous moments or, in some instances, the complete break-down of the interview.

Delaying. There are points in the therapeutic process when the helper, for any of a variety of reasons, does not wish to make a direct reply to the client or believes that the pace of the encounter needs to be slowed down. Delaying responses serve an extremely useful purpose at such moments. These techniques are usually very simple and may consist of a repetition of the question the client has asked, a request for amplification or clarification, or any plausible phrase or gesture that gives the practitioner a few seconds to consider a reply or to deflect the client's immediate concern.

Blurring. At similar points the therapist may believe that it will better serve the immediate purposes of engagement if a reply to a client's query is broadly and generally phrased; hence the em-ployment of deliberately generalized or blurred responses. Often these are times when in the clinician's judgment the emotional intensity of the moment has reached a height which is detrimental and a blurred response can be helpful in reducing this emotional arousal. Any reader desiring an example of this technique need only observe a typical interview with a politician to appreciate that even the most specific question can be given a vague yet plausible reply. As therapists we like to believe that our purposes and motivations are loftier than those of politicians, yet the intent of blurring techniques is the same—to avoid potential entangle-ments through a deliberately generalized reply.

Deferring. This technique consists of *agreeing with,* rather than challenging, client statements and is usually employed where there is clear indication that the potential client is reluctant or ambivalent about professional intervention or where there is a need to avoid direct confrontation at an early stage of the initial interview. Thus the therapist's comments are intended to implicitly convey the message that the client's independence or freedom of opinion or choice will be respected. For example, an individual might present his difficulties as minor and, rather than dispute this viewpoint, the clinician might defer to the client by openly agreeing that this could be true.

Thus, in an initial interview, a thirty-year-old Vietnam veteran told how his family had insisted that he seek treatment because of depression. However, he vehemently declared that he was "no more depressed than anyone else." The clinician accepted this position without dispute and asked the client to describe "this everyday depression you're going through." Deferred to rather than challenged, the client readily entered into an exposition of a number of stressful life problems, including an understandable degree of depression.

Embedding. In working with troubled people there are moments when the clinician believes that it would be helpful to suggest a different viewpoint to the client but anticipates that the client is likely to discount or challenge this position. For example, optimistic redefinitions of aspects of the client's difficulties or normalizing statements with positive implications, if directly delivered, can be strongly disputed or deprecated by a pessimistic client. At other times the therapist may want to create a positive climate within the session without appearing obviously reassuring to the client. The technique of embedding is especially useful for such strategic purposes (Bandler et al., 1976).

Embedding consists of placing a key statement within the context of one or more statements of a less significant nature. The technique is frequently used in hypnotic inductions, where the therapist will embed suggestions for relaxation or calmness within a monotonous or irrelevant patter. Thus a client with difficulties in coping with a job may describe her discouragement with this situation but at the same time contend that her problems are largely the result of unfair demands by her supervisor. The therapist may wish to challenge this fixed viewpoint but, at an engagement stage, might be concerned about alienating the client. This could be managed by an embedded response:

Therapist: You must get awfully worn down and angry as you go through these pressures, day after day. That feeling of being unfairly treated can really get at you, and I guess you must almost have to fight at times to keep from looking at everything that way. The frustration can get so strong when you're caught in a real trap like this.

Embedded within this response is a suggestion, "You must almost have to fight at times to keep from looking at everything that way," which is intended to convey the possibility that the client's current belief system is playing a part in her difficulties. Like many of the engagement techniques described, embedding is intended, not to evoke an immediate change, but through cumulative repetition to create a climate in which varied possibilities can be considered. The objective, of course, is to offer a more functional alternative to the narrow or fixed beliefs and behaviors that have proved unworkable for the troubled client.

Stages of the Initial Interview

Harry Stack Sullivan discusses many of the nuances of the initial interview in his book *The Psychiatric Interview* (1954). This neglected classic of the therapeutic art can be profitably read and reread by the practicing clinician of any discipline or theoretical persuasion. Although he ostensibly is addressing himself to the psychiatrist, Sullivan is careful to point our that his examination of the interpersonal process of interviewing has broad applications. He notes:

In referring to the interviewee or client, I shall sometimes speak of him as the patient, but I imply no restriction of the relevance of what I say to the medical field, believing that, for the most part, it will apply equally well to the fields of social work or personnel management, for example [p. 4].

Sullivan identifies four stages within the therapeutic interview. These will form a useful framework for examining the process. However, in the context of brief therapy I will place a somewhat different emphasis than Sullivan on certain aspects of each of these phases. In contrast to the objectives outlined in the previous chapter, this delineation of phases within the initial interview is intended to give the practitioner a sense of the ongoing and inter-related process of this first meeting. Four stages are suggested:

1. Inception
2. Reconnaisance
3. Detailed inquiry
4. Interruption or termination

In the succeeding sections of this chapter each phase will be briefly defined and its major characteristics discussed in some detail. Many of the engagement techniques discussed earlier (and the major goals outlined in Chapter 4) are related to particular phases of this process.

THE INCEPTION PHASE

This refers, of course, to the first few moments of the interview and, as Sullivan (1954) notes, "includes the formal reception of the person who comes to be interviewed and an inquiry about, or a reference to, the circumstances of his coming" (p. 37). The inception phase should also incorporate some reference to what-ever information the therapist has been given about the potential client and establish a reasonable purpose for the session. These beginning moments are often awkward and uncomfortable for both therapist and client. Perhaps because of this discomfort the inception phase, despite its great importance, has been particu-larly neglected in the clinical literature.

Prior the the literal moment when client and therapist first meet, both are, obviously, unrelated individuals, one of whom is experiencing some sort of difficulty in life while the other is presumed to possess a special knowledge and skill in dealing with such problems. The beginning of therapy then brings together two human beings whose immediate characteristics may (or may not) result in their continuing to meet. If they continue their relationship, for whatever length of time, both client and clinician hope that these encounters will be beneficial to the client. Furthermore, the practitioner expects that the relationship will offer a gratifying opportunity to utilize the expertise that he or she has acquired in a chosen profession.

The outcome of any initial interview is at best a chancy matter. In a case example given in Chapter 1 I described a pregnant young woman whose boyfriend was in jail and whose immediate family were caught up in their own concerns. Unable to find assistance within her natural social networks, she felt concerned about how to cope with a number of financial, emotional, and practical issues over the next few months of her life. A medical social worker, at the suggestion of another professional, interviewed the young woman to offer help. Despite this juxtaposition of a person in need of help and a practitioner able to offer assistance, one might still question whether a viable relationship will occur. Will this woman reappear for further interviews, if these are planned? Or will she, like many other potential clients, drop from sight and never receive the benefits counseling might have offered?

All of these statements may sound quite mundane and hardly worth discussion. Yet it is well to remember that the *potential* relationship of helper and client, described above, does not usually continue for more than an extremely short time. The findings on premature termination or early drop-out tell us bleakly that only one of three clients will be seen after the initial interview and that hardly one of five will continue for more than a very few sessions. In other words, the critical problem of the initial interview is one of engagement—the clinician has about an hour to reverse the strong probability that the person being seen is not going to return or will do so for only a very few sessions. As there is no reason to believe that the clients who drop out are different, in type or degree of difficulty, from those who continue (Baekland and Lundwall, 1975; Garfield, 1971, 1980), there is good reason to carefully examine these early moments of the helping relationship. It is here that the clinician has an opportunity to begin to influence the relationship in such a way as to increase the probability of the client's returning and benefiting from professional help. Indeed, as the data indicate that time is extremely limited, it is apparent that the therapist must utilize it fully if an effective relationship is to be established.*

In considering these beginning moments, it is useful to remember the many differences between a social relationship and a therapeutic relationship and, in particular, the differing conventions governing the conversation that takes place in each of these contexts. There are any number of rules, mainly unwritten, that govern the conduct of social conversations between comparative strangers. From the social perspective, for example, one does not ask questions of a highly personal nature such as ''How are you and your wife getting along sexually?'' or make such plainspoken statements as ''There must be times when you wish he wasn't even your child,'' which challenge the other's motivations. If an individual becomes emotionally upset during a social conversation, conventional expressions of sympathy are expected, and it would be considered tactless to respond in such a way as to highlight or increase an individual's distress. All of these conventions, and more, will soon be broken in therapeutic conversation.

In order to make the transition from the social to the therapeutic context in the least jarring manner, it is often helpful if the therapist deliberately encourages a few moments of social conversation at the beginning of the initial meeting. This does not

---

*None of the foregoing discussion is intended to convey that every person who asks for help *must* become a client or that there are not a number of people who benefit from very brief contact. However, careful attention to the management of the initial interview will enable those individuals who decide against continuing to make this choice under the best of circumstances. Further, those who need only a very brief period of help will similarly benefit from a skillful handling of the first contact.

have to be a particularly scintillating exchange, and indeed it is often of a pedestrian nature. For example, the helper may inquire about the weather or ask the client if parking was easily available. This social exchange gives the therapist an opportunity to greet the client by name and shake hands, indicate where he can hang up his coat and where he should sit, and carry out any other small amenities that may be useful to the client at this potentially anxious moment.

Moreover, the social aspects of the conversation, however forced, serve several other valuable purposes. It must be remembered that the client is entering into alien territory and, at a minimum, deserves some small chance to orient himself. In the unfamiliar confines of the clinician's office it can be not only a courtesy but a minor relief to be told, for instance, where to sit. Similar inquiries about whether the client wishes to smoke and, if so, furnishing an ashtray add to the sense of being welcomed and made comfortable. These fleeting gestures are a part of the social ritual of greeting and by their familiar ring can ease at least a portion of the client's uneasiness about what may lie ahead. In other words, the social aspects of the inception phase serve as a transition into the therapeutic relationship and, like all transitions, attempt to make a change from one state to another less perceptible or uncomfortable.

Such family therapy advocates as Haley (1976) and Minuchin (1974) have written about the socializing techniques of the first session. Minuchin characterizes the therapist as "host" during these moments, making the conventional but reassuring gestures of welcome, while Haley speaks of this phase as an opportunity for both practitioner and client to observe each other.

I find this latter aspect particularly useful. The client is unknown to me as I am to him, and even a few moments of observation, cloaked by the social conventions, can frequently give me a beginning sense of the individual I am about meet. What does he look like? How is he dressed? How is this potential client handling himself at this very moment? A frown, for example, can indicate discomfort or suspicion, a trembling hand may suggest a person in acute stress, and so on. All of these clues are extremely tentative, of course, and usually require no immediate comment, but they can be helpful in orienting the clinician to what may lie ahead.

As these few moments of social conversation draw to a close, the need for transition to the therapeutic conversation appears, and the burden of making this shift falls upon the therapist. Unless the client has literally walked in off the street, the therapist usually has a general notion of the problem he or she is experiencing. This knowledge can be used as a part of the bridge needed to lead into the therapeutic discourse that will occupy the remainder of the initial session. Such a transitional statement by the practitioner can take the following form:

> From what I understood when we talked on the telephone, your're quite concerned with some problems you're meeting to do with anxiety and stress in your life and finding these hard to deal with. I realize that you may be feeling uncomfortable and edgy right now in talking to me, because I'm very much a stranger to you and I know it isn't easy to talk about personal problems. See if you can give me a better idea of what's concerning you and let's spend this next hour that we have trying to decide if the kind of counseling I can offer would be helpful to you. Just start wherever you want and if there are things I don't follow I'll ask some questions.

A very similar emphasis on this sort of transitional statement of practitioner understanding and purpose is discussed in Ewing's (1978) monograph on crisis intervention and in Schulman's (1979) brilliant examination of helping skills. Schulman suggests that the clinician "must attempt to clarify the purpose of the meeting by a simple, nonjargonized, and direct statement" (p. 29). He sees such openness as closely related to (and clearly anticipating) the contracting about purpose and goals that must take place between helper and client later in the initial interview.

It must be emphasized that the therapist's statement presented above is a planned attempt to influence certain aspects of the ensuing process in a way that will make engagement and the initiation of brief treatment more likely. It contains a number of facets that I believe play some part in the continuing process of engagement and deserve further comment.

At the very beginning of the statement, for example, the clinician is attempting to give the potential client a brief version of what she knows about the client's difficulties. If the locus of the problem is more specifically known, this could be stated: "I understand you're very concerned about your marriage." In any case, the therapist keeps this part of the statement brief and in effect regards it as a starting point, subject to further amplification and correction, form which the client can proceed. I try to capture some aspect of emotional disturbance in this capsule statement of problem as I want to suggest from the very beginning of the helping process that I am interested in emotions and will be frequently responding to this dimension of the client's life.

A similar emphasis on emotion appears in the next sentence as the clinician suggests that the client may be uncomfortable at this very moment. This is, once again, an effort to highlight the emotional dimension and to convey the therapist's willingness to address this issue directly. One might characterize this as "easy empathy" in the sense that almost anyone in the situation of being a potential client in a mental health or social service setting is likely to be experiencing some degree of discomfort. Thus the practitioner is able to demonstrate, with minimal effort, a degree of understanding that can begin to accumulate toward this major goal of the engagement process.

The time limits of the initial session are spelled out through the therapist's comment on "this next hour," and it is suggested that some sort of agreement about further counseling may be possible by the end of this time. My preference is to state this possibility in a tentative (yet positive) manner as at this point I have little idea whether the prospective client is eagerly seeking help or has come in only under the utmost duress. This is not to say that the therapist's conviction that counseling is highly useful to people has to be concealed; it simply recognizes that not everyone is immediately ready to grasp at this possibility. Deferring to the client's possible reluctance in advance can save the helper from some difficult moments.

Finally, it will be noted that there is a frequent use of the personal pronoun throughout the helper's transitional statement. This, again, is a deliberate emphasis. The therapist expects that the client will talk personally and openly during the ensuing interview, and although actual therapist self-disclosure may not be appropriate at this opening point, the least the clinician can do is to suggest her own involvement through such a choice of phrasing. This offers the client a minimal model for disclosure and is one of many attempts on the part of the clinician to increase the probablility of more favorable outcomes.

THE RECONNAISANCE PHASE

Sullivan (1954) suggests that within this stage of the initial interview the clinician is "concerned with trying to get some notion of the person's identity—who he is and how he happens to get to be the person who has come to the office" (pp. 37–38). Sullivan speaks of the objective of this phase in terms of obtaining "a rough outline of the social and personal history of the patient" (p. 37). In short-term treatment, however, I believe that the reconnaisance is most usefully visualized as a time when the client is actively encouraged to describe how he or she views the difficulties that have led to this initial meeting. The therapist does not gather any formal history, but concentrates on responding to the client's immediate statements. But throughout this description there will be a number of points where the clinician may ask pertinent questions in order to clarify aspects of the client's life that are not obvious from his or her statements.

Care should be exercised to avoid questions that are not essential to the concentrated focus of short-term treatment. For example, as Mr. Faber (see Chapter 3) described his difficulties in relationships with women and indicated that his parents had been moralistic and inhibiting about sexuality, it was not necessary to ask for many details of his early history. The issue of *how* his family had had this effect upon him was not important, although the need for sexual reeducation in an accepting atmosphere became an immediate hypothesis for possible intervention.

As I pointed out in discussing the inception phase of the therapeutic encounter, the movement into the reconnaisance stage is stimulated by the practitioner's summary statement of the immediate objectives of the initial session. A few clients may query or challenge this statement, particularly if it runs drastically counter to their expectations, but most simply launch into an exposition of the difficulties in life that are currently troubling them. The manner and content of this beginning description vary, of course, from one person to another, along any number of dimensions. The series of initial interviews presented in Davenloo's (1978) *Short-Term Dynamic Psychotherapy* run the gamut of these differing presentations of self. These and other examples drawn from practice will offer illustrations.

Some people immediately begin to talk about themselves and the particularly bothersome emotions they are experiencing:

"Well the last few months I've been very depressed and I started to have tantrums because I felt so burdened mentally" [p. 201].*

Others speak of impelling actions:

"I just want to run away from everything, just leave the city, and go away by myself" [p. 100].

The beginning focus may be terse and factual:

The only thing that bothers me is that I've always got headaches and pains in my head" [pp. 277–278].

For some prospective clients the emphasis may be on the actions of other people:

*Page numbers after client statements refer to quotations from the Davenloo (1978) interview transcripts.

"My husband's drinking himself to death and he won't do a damn thing about it."

Some individuals are vague and apparently unfocused:

"I feel lost; I feel like I don't have a center. I feel out of touch with myself" [p. 247].

Or the client's initial expression of difficulty may touch on an important aspect of social functioning:

"I've been having this fear of being out on the street, and then it developed into being afraid of being at work—not all the time, just some days" [p. 225].

Finally, there may be little the individual seemingly wants for himself as he grudgingly approaches counseling:

"They said I had to come here or I was going to get fired from my job."

Whatever direction the client's beginning thrust into problem expression may take, the practitioner's concern during this early phase largely centers on the question "Who is this person and what is troublesome at present in his or her life?" Three major therapist activities predominate and intermingle throughout the reconaissance.

First, the therapist must look for every opportunity to respond empathically to the prospective client's immediate emotions. As I have previously noted, this should be done in the plainest of language, avoiding technical terms and attempting to respond to the full intensity of the feelings that the client directly or indirectly is expressing.

Helpers sometimes hesitate to recognize the depth of emotion the client is experiencing and consequently detract from this powerful relationship bond. Such hesitation is sometimes rationalized on the grounds that clients are "not ready" to have their emotions explicitly identified or that a forthright acknowledgment of turmoil or despair could somehow worsen their situation. Empathic response, as I noted earlier, attempts to recognize the emotions clients are plainly expressing or that are clearly part of the experience they are undergoing. There is unlikely to be any harm in directly acknowledging, for example, that the client who is directly expressing anger is angry or in suggesting that someone who is undergoing a serious illness or a divorce may be anxious or frightened. Empathic response is not an attempt to probe into the client or to *interpret* his or her emotions, but, most fundamentally, a persistent effort to establish a human connection with the client's pain or dissatisfaction with life.

Second, the process of problem identification has begun in a significant way in this early phase of contact, and the helper must carefully attend to the client's perspective on this central issue. The essential question is very simple: "What major problems in living is this person experiencing at this moment?"

As the client tells his or her story, the aspects of life that are most dissatisfying will begin to unfold. With many people this expression of difficulty does not suggest an individual ready to take an active and perceptive role in the process of change. Feelings of helplessness or doubt, projection onto others or self-blame may permeate the client's account. The clinician, however, makes little effort at this point to explore any single problem in depth or to challenge the client's viewpoint. In large part the clinician's concern is to encourage clients to range across their current life in an effort to describe its most troubling aspects. It can be helpful, at this point, for the clinician to make a brief written list of the major areas of concern as the client describes them. This should simply summarize each problem ("You're concerned about your child's bedwetting" or "You and your husband have a lot of difficulty in agreeing about how to discipline the children"), and the list, as it is composed, should be frequently shared with the client for revision and amplification.

Finally, the therapist must consciously make some beginning efforts to build hope in order to provide some foundation for the problem negotiation and contracting that will take place in the later stages of the interview. At this stage of the interview only the most tentative ventures can be made in this vital area, but they

must be attempted. Ripple et al. (1964) underscored the exquisitely balanced interaction between hope and distress and the critical relationship of this balance to continuance in treatment in
Motivation, Capacity and Opportunity, their classic study of the
early phases of the helping process:

> The client's discomfort and his hope regarding a solution of the
> problems are in the foreground in his initial help-seeking. Regard-
> less of the specifics of goal or service sought or the capacities
> available for use, it is the motivating pressure that provides the
> dynamic for engagement in problem solving or in using the help-
> ing offered [p. 206].

The arousal of hope was discussed in the preceding chapter as
one of the primary goals of the initial interview. Few clinicians
would disagree with this emphasis, but some perplexing questions
arise. How can one make what is said in an effort to elicit hope during the engagement process sound like more than a pious desire or
an empty piece of rhetoric? What specific activities on the part of the
therapist can be employed to build the sort of positive expectation
in the client that will enhance engagement and, further, form a
beginning basis for change? A number of strategies and techniques have already been suggested, earlier in this chapter, that
can assist in eliciting hopefulness. Thus redefinitions are utilized
to suggest a more positive viewpoint toward perceived difficulties, or normalizing strategies are employed to convey to the
client that a particular problem is not uncommon. At the same
time, the clinician does not attempt to promote an unrealistically
positive atmosphere. Some edge of anxiety or dissatisfaction can
be a useful motivation for seeking change.

During the reconnaisance stage the clinician listens for any
indication on the client's part that the difficulties being described
are not what he or she wants from life. Whatever the intensity of
negative emotion or negative belief expressed, is the client conveying something about attempts, however feeble or misdirected,
to master these forces? Such tentative practitioner efforts at enhancing hope can often be reinforced by empathic response—

"You sound terribly discouraged about managing these problems with your daughter, but I get the idea that you don't want your life together to just go on like this." In effect, the therapist's intervention is directed toward mobilizing the client's sense of self-efficacy through these preliminary suggestions that the immediate dilemma has a solution other than resignation or despair.

THE DETAILED INQUIRY

In many initial interviews the movement from the reconnaissance phase into the detailed inquiry may be almost imperceptible. Its overall goal is to increase the information available to both clinician and client. Thus at this point in the interview the clinician makes a deliberate effort to expand upon the nature and degree of the difficulties in living that the client has described. As Sullivan (1954) points out, much of the detailed inquiry "is a matter of improving upon earlier approximations of understanding" (p. 90) and at times may involve a radical change in the impressions the clinician initially obtained. The helper may also inquire about important relationships or potential problem areas that the client's previous description had not covered. In initiating short-term treatment, it is at this stage that the therapist begins the important process of negotiation that will determine the prospective focus and goals of treatment. During this part of the detailed inquiry the client learns more specifically about the potential nature of the helping process.

In essence, then, the two essential tasks for client and the helper during the detailed inquiry are *clarification* and *negotiation*. The problems that the client has identified during the preceding conversation need to be examined in greater detail, and client and therapist must engage in negotiation as to whether they will work together on one or two of these problems in an ongoing therapeutic relationship.

The helper should not feel compelled to examine each of the client's problems in their complete complexity. The therapist must *selectively* explore, and once again, a deliberate process of simplification is apparent. That is to say, the objective of the detailed inquiry stage is to fill in gaps and clarify aspects of the client's earlier presentation that have puzzled the clinician.

Most of this exploration is sharply focused on the client's current relationships and living situation. Historical material is seldom gathered in depth unless it has an immediate relevance to the problems in living being discussed. Thus with Mr. Jurecko and Mrs. Lorenson (see Chapter 3), practically all of the initial exploration concentrated on their current life and their problems of major concern. Limiting exploration so drastically may require a leap of faith for the therapist inexperienced in brief treatment, as conventional training has tended to emphasize a detailed exploration of almost every facet of the potential client's past and current life. Indeed, there was an era when all practitioners were taught to spend six to eight interviews in assessment and relationship-building activities—a period of time equivalent to the totality of a great many brief treatment encounters.

Helpers may find it useful to follow a formal schedule of inquiry during this phase and ask the client about such areas as job, education, financial circumstances, social relationships, family, and marriage. Aspects of each of these dimensions of living may have been touched on earlier but may still require clarification. Others may not have been mentioned, and in such instances the practitioner will conduct a brief probe in order to elicit needed information. The tendency of the short-term therapist is to inquire directly about such possibly relevant connections but to accept the client's assessment concerning whether a given area is problematic or nonproblematic. An extensive exploration is not attempted unless the therapist has urgent reason to believe that this is necessary.

Perhaps even more important than the selective expansion on life difficulties is the question of problem priority. If a client is contending with four or five problems, which is the most meaningful? Which problem does the client most wish to solve? Therapists can place different values on living than their clients, and it is best to ask the client specifically for such an assessment. For example, in a case I supervised the clinician was surprised to find that a young adult woman placed greater emphasis on working out some moderately distressing difficulties in her immediate social relationships than on grappling with a troublesome relationship with her mother. As the two areas were only peripherally related (theoretical views to the contrary), progress on the first area was quite feasible even while the other conflict remained unchanged. In general the practitioner in brief treatment is well advised to respect the client's wishes in matters of problem priority unless there is a strongly compelling reason to suggest shifting to another focus. The predictive powers of most of our available theoretical frameworks are not sufficiently accurate to justify this sort of shift except in a minority of cases.

The actual mechanics of prioritizing problems can be managed fairly easily if the helper has been tracking the client's difficulties by formulating a written list. I often ask the client to read through this list, reflect on the impact of each problem area, and numerically rate the problems from most to least pressing. This is usually an appropriate time to offer some explanatory structuring to the effect that the best problem solving takes place when one selects a single, important problem and concentrates on its resolution.

However, whatever the practitioner may be thinking about the problems the client is experiencing or the potential help that therapeutic intervention might offer, it is necessary to elicit the client's views. The work of Arnold Lazare and his colleagues (1972, 1975a, 1975b) offers a number of empirically grounded guidelines for managing this aspect of the initial interview. They point out that the concept of the patient or client's *request* has been confused with the related but different notion of *expectation:*

Expectations . . . represent the *anticipation* of roles, techniques, duration of treatment, and outcome. These expectations may be based on wishes, fears, or even stories from friends. Requests, on the other hand, represent hopes or desires [Lazare et al., 1972, p. 873].

Thus, in contrast to his or her expectation of what counseling will be like or how the therapist will act, the request represents what the client wants to gain from therapy. For example, a prospective client may *expect* that her difficulties will be met with scepticism or even blame from the unknown practitioner whom she is about to meet. On the other hand, her *request* (or hope) might be that she be given some useful advice on how to deal with the problems or an opportunity to release the pent-up feelings they have engendered.

Expectation and request may coincide or may be dramatically different. The Lazare group's work has substantiated the prevalence of misunderstanding and confusion between clinician and client when the request is not directly obtained, and in relation to this task the group has identified fourteen specific categories into which client requests commonly fall. These can be grouped around four major themes (Lazare et al., 1972):

1. *Be a supportive person.* The requests here are for control, reality contact, succorance, institutional support, confession, ventilation, and advice. The researchers carefully differentiate each of these requests and offer some cogent clinical guidelines on the quality and quantity of therapist activity each requires.

2. *Be a psychotherapist.* Within this overall category the individual may be requesting clarification about pressing internal conflicts or, more specifically, help with immediate personal and interpersonal change. Further research on client requests (Burgoyne et al., 1979) has found that low socioeconomic clients often make such requests but frequently combine them with requests in other categories. It also found that because of the prevailing belief that people in the low socioeconomic group desire only concrete services or direct advice, clinicians have real difficulty in distinguishing their more therapeutic requests and appropriately responding.

3. *Be an authority figure.* Here the potential client is hoping to enlist the organizational, administrative, or social intervention powers of the helping person in relation to the problems being experienced. The client may believe, quite legitimately, that

some specific service at the helper's command can offer relief. For example, the individual may envisage the clinician as a potential advocate in dealing with another agency or institution or may wish to obtain a concrete resource that the practitioner controls. Helpers of all disciplines should be careful not to neglect or deprecate such intervention.

4. *Miscellaneous requests.* These are usually concerned with direction or referral to a more appropriate helping source (Lazare calls this "community triage"). For a small but significant group, literally *nothing* is desired. Individuals in this latter group usually have been pressured or compelled to ask for help.

Lazare and his colleagues (1975a) suggest that the request be elicited about midway through the initial interview. This allows enough time for rapport to develop yet leaves sufficient leeway for client and therapist to negotiate, if the request is inappropriate. They offer some specific guidelines:

> We have been most successful in eliciting the patient request by asking, "How do you hope (or wish) I (or the clinic) can help?" The questions "What do you want?" or "What do you expect?" should be avoided as they are likely to be perceived as a confrontation. The words "wish" or "hope," in contrast, give the patient permission to state requests he does not necessarily expect will be granted . . . . When the request has finally been stated and elaborated, it is important that the clinician acknowledge that he has heard and understood the request. Otherwise, the patient may wonder whether the clinician heard the request, was offended by it, or didn't believe it worthy of a response [p. 554].

Understanding the client's request plays an important role in the process of contracting. The goal of contracting is for client and helper to arrive at an open decision whether to work together, in a clearly understood way, on a particular client problem. The contracting process, in this third stage of the first interview, becomes a matter of reconciling client request and therapist judgment in relation to how to work on the problem area that has been selected for attention. If client request and clinical judgment are reasonably close, then arriving at a contract is relatively straightforward. If there are discrepancies, however, negotiation must take place. It is then up to the therapist to explain, for example, how it might be more beneficial to the client to learn how to be assertive than merely to ventilate the feelings aroused by humiliating social relationships.

A clear agreement to work together on a specific problem is one of the hallmarks of professional helping and is an essential legitimization of the change strategies the therapist may employ at later stages in the helping process. Asking clients to disclose intimate aspects of their life, requesting task performance, confronting discrepancies between client verbalization and behavior, and so on are justifiable only in the context of such an agreement.

A final issue deserves some consideration. As the detailed inquiry begins, the therapist is faced with the decision as to whether the goals of the initial interview can be met within a single session. If the client's exposition of his or her major problems is still so fragmentary and unclear that detailed inquiry is hardly possible, it is obvious that more time will be required. Second, if motivation is extremely low or if the client is plainly responding only to external pressures in seeking help, then the possibility of a viable contract may appear remote. In such instances the clinician may decide to devote the remainder of the interview to problem exploration or to attempts to enhance the relationship, contracting for a further session to conclude the usual goals of the first interview.*

INTERRUPTION OR TERMINATION

In the final stage of the initial interview the helper plays an active role in bringing the interview to a conclusion. This may

---

*In such situations some clinicians will contract for four to six interviews to explore the client's difficulties. My preference is to avoid the vagueness or indecision this can sometimes promote by contracting for only a *single* further session. This strategy is an attempt to maintain the pressures of an explicit time limit and in addition to continue a concentrated focus on specific problem identification.

represent an actual end of contact between helper and client or an interruption in a process that will resume again. In either case there are certain actions that the therapist can take that will consolidate the termination or, on the other hand, enhance the probability of the client's return if further contact is planned.

If the participants have arrived at a problem focus and have contracted to work together, then the therapist must set a time limit and define an initial task (along with any other unsettled details such as next appointment time or fee). Where a further interview has been negotiated in order to complete the engagement process, these tasks can usually be deferred to the next session. On the other hand, as Sullivan (1954) notes, the initial interview may represent a termination of contact with the client. For some a referral to a more suitable agency or clinic may have been arranged; for others it may not have been possible to negotiate a viable helping contract.

Setting time limits merits some further discussion. Practitioners unfamiliar with short-term intervention seem to have the notion that the setting of time limits is an exact science. Experienced short-term therapists, on the other hand, are exasperatingly casual about this process and sometimes almost inarticulate about why, for instance, ten sessions were stipulated with a certain client rather than eight or twelve. However, some aspects of the concept of time limits are quite clear. The basic position of most brief therapists is that time limits must be of a foreseeable length, and that the exact nature of the time limit should be firmly and confidently explained to the client during the one or two interviews of the engagement process.

Beyond this it is difficult to ascertain how the brief therapist determines the limit. In some cases a research project (Reid and Shyne, 1969) or simply an accustomed way of working (Mann, 1973) determines that every case will be offered a set number of interviews. Other therapists follow an agency policy that predetermines the number of sessions (Jacobson, 1965; Leventhal and Weinberger, 1975). Certain change procedures—sexual therapy (Masters and Johnson, 1970) for example—suggest an expected number of interviews. Some therapists rely on entirely subjective guidelines and will say, "I'll suggest eight sessions if the problems look easy and twelve to fifteen sessions if they look hard." The same therapists will further confuse the picture by prescribing, say six rather than ten sessions for a particular client because they believe that the shorter time limit will be more acceptable to the client.

Brief therapists are usually quite direct and matter of fact in stipulating time limits to their clients and often use this as a means of embedding a hopeful message: "I think we should work together for no longer than ten sessions, and this should be enough to help you feel much more capable in managing your children." Another important dynamic, as I noted in the preceding chapter, is the fact that the therapist does not negotiate the length of the contract with the client, but assumes this responsibility as a function of his professional role. Implicitly this tends to convey that the clinician, as an expert in interpersonal relationships, believes that progress is possible within this time. Negotiating the time limit could suggest that the therapist is simply being solicitous about not inconveniencing the client. Such inappropriate deferral could tend to weaken the hope and confidence that firm time setting can potentially inspire.

Similarly, task assignment appears to be a highly subjective matter in many respects; therapists inexperienced in brief therapy seek exact guidelines and seasoned practitioners tend to be rather casual. Like time limits, moreover, task assignment appears to be importantly influenced by such therapist factors as firmness and confidence and additionally by the need to present the client with a plausible rationale for action. As I pointed out in Chapter 4, most early tasks are attempts to gain further information about the nature and degree of the client's problem or, in a very minor way, serve as a stimulus toward activity. There is no reason that either of these rationales cannot be explained to the client, and this is usually sufficient structuring to promote client cooperation in task performance. Despite reports in the clinical literature in which the therapist immediately devises an ingenious task sufficient to almost magically propel the client into adequate functioning, the bulk of tasks in actual practice are quite pedestrian. Chapter 7 will discuss many of the theoretical and technical issues in task assignment in greater detail.

Finally, as Sullivan (1954) notes, the initial interview may represent a termination of contact with the client. For some a referral to a more appropriate agency may be needed. With others it may not have been possible to work out a feasible contract. In either case the helper has an obligation, I believe, to try to pull together the conclusions that have been reached in the session. Reviewing with the client the reasons that referral to another agency has been suggested and the benefits the client may gain from this can significantly enhance the possibility of follow-through. Weisman (1976) outlines an even more active technology for referral, which he calls "linkage," on the grounds that data from empirical studies (Ryan, 1969) indicate that hardly one out of four referred clients actually reaches the other helping source. A similar review can be carried out even where therapist and client have decided not to continue further interviews. This is often in the form of a summary by the practitioner of his or her understanding of the client's difficulties and, where appropriate, a frank recognition of the reasons why the client does not want (or need) continued professional help.

Chapter 6

Challenging Stereotyped Description: Behavior Enactment

The thing is recovered from familiarity by means of an exercise in familiarity.

—Walker Percy

Although seemingly dissimilar in theoretical orientation and therapeutic goals, behavioral therapy and psychodrama have both made frequent use of deliberate enactments of real-life events— past, present, and future—as a vehicle for learning and change. Whether we call such dramatized vignettes "simulations," "role-plays," or "behavior rehearsal," their essential commonality, I believe, is the attempt to change the therapeutic situation from a conversation of a peculiar sort, an interview, into a miniature replication of a fragment of the client's life.

Behavior enactment and rehearsal methods offer the helper a powerful medium for change, with the potentiality to move beyond exclusively verbal efforts to describe problematic or conflicted life situations into a visual and physical dimension. The attempt to portray the client's actual or anticipated behavior in any troublesome encounter can stimulate a novel awareness of inhibiting attitudes or beliefs. Even though the simulation itself has certain limitations, it can reveal the arousal of dysfunctional emotion or display deficits in life skills more vividly than verbal discussion alone can.

Clinical writers from the most diverse theoretical backgrounds have contributed to this viewpoint. Thus such family therapists as Minuchin (1967, 1974, 1978) have contended that is is futile even to attempt to understand the patterned, often ritualized dance of the family through descriptions which, at best, are secondhand. From an entirely different theoretical orientation, gestalt therapists (Hatcher and Himelstein, 1976) have devised any number of ingenious therapeutic permutations (the "empty chair" technique, for example) intended to transport the individual beyond the boundaries of ordinary experience into realms where the unexpected may emerge or where hidden aspects of self can be viewed.

Behavioral therapists (Bandura, 1977b) have become almost contemptuous, at times, of the efficacy of "talk therapy" to influence the course of human thoughts, behavior, and emotions and have strongly advocated the employment of direct observation and performance methods. Finally, J. L. Moreno's (1959) pioneering development of the enactment methods of psychodrama represents a major contribution to the efforts to find ways of moving beyond the tyranny of words.

Paul Wachtel (1977), in his integrative work on therapeutic practice, *Psychoanalysis and Behavior Therapy*, points out the need for methods of enabling the client to transfer the learnings of therapy into the outside world:

> Without explicit efforts to bridge the gap between the nurturant therapy relationship and the more demanding world outside, there is a good chance that the patient will learn to discriminate and act one way with the therapist and another with everyone else. The therapist then has the conviction—correct as far as his (in-session) direct experience of the patient is concerned—that the patient has become freer, more open, more healthy and genuine; yet in the patient's day-to-day living, change is far less extensive [p. 232].

Wachtel suggests that for many clients change can take place more rapidly if there is an opportunity, through enactments of various kinds, to build new relationship patterns. The very difficulties of the troubled or inhibited person may have "limited the possibility of his observing and assimilating how people behave in various situations" (p. 233). Even though the individual, in a broad sense, "knows" what to do, this knowledge may not be particularly usable under the real demands of living. As Wachtel comments, "The patient may be able to describe what is called for, but not to put it into practice" (p.233).

In his discussion of role-playing and rehearsal methods Wachtel emphasizes their utility, not only in building social and interpersonal skills but as an integral part of the assessment process:

> Role-playing procedures are also of value in giving the therapist a picture of the patient's style in a way which no amount of description of the "So then I said that I didn't like what he was doing" variety can convey.... One discovers something in seeing the patient actually play out just what he said and how he said it that is masked in the patient's reporting of the event [p. 234].

Some of the reluctance of clients to role-play comes from this very fear of exposing themselves to a scrutiny which might have been easily avoided by a purely descriptive statement. Although he cautions the helper against absolutely insisting on the client's role playing, Wachtel also points out how the client, though initially hesitant, may benefit from an enhanced understanding of self in real-life interaction, even from a feared enactment. He also stresses that the role reversal that takes place in some types of simulation can frequently build client awareness of the other person's feelings or of the client's own impact on his interpersonal world. Wachtel comments:

> When the therapist models the way the patient *has* acted, the patient can be helped to understand his impact on the other person; when the therapist models how the patient *might* act, the patient

may gain some insight into himself, into what he is on the verge of feeling inclined to do [p. 237].

Corsini's (1966) discussion of role-playing techniques in psychotherapy is one of the most complete accounts of this medium of change. He points our that role-playing methods are "generally based on the inductive principle; one learns complex matters best from unit behaviors which lead to generalization" (p. 33).

Three major theoretical constructs support the utilization of role playing or (in the terminology employed in this book) behavior enactment:

1. *Simultaneity.* In Corsini's view the greatest theoretical advantage of role playing is its capacity to elicit the full range of cognitive, affective, and behavioral elements contained in a problematic situation. Not only can significant aspects of thinking, feeling, and acting be concurrently exhibited and experienced in the enactment, but, as Corsini points out, "due to the summating effects of each on the other, they tend to be heightened—exaggerated—forced to fuller limits" (p. 13).

2. *Spontaneity.* Corsini defines spontaneity as "natural, rapid, unforced, self-generated behavior in new situations" (p. 13) and suggests that enactment methods can tap this potential reservoir within the individual. He acknowledges that although it would undoubtedly be better if the client could simply attempt new behaviors in real life, this is often unlikely. Behavior rehearsal offers a protected opportunity for unexpected capacities to emerge. At the same time, the client's self-protective tendencies, so often exhibited through censored or prevaricating verbal description, are less likely to be operative.

3. *Veridicality.* Corsini compares role-playing experiences to the simulated training apparatuses employed in airplane pilot instruction. Although the participant knows that the apparatus, or the enactment, is not real it can assume a subjective or psychological reality. Much of this depends upon the attitude of the clinician, who must convey a sense of confidence that, within under-

standable limits, behavior rehearsal can capture many of the nuances of real life. At the same time the helper should be careful not to oversell the method, but should clearly recognize its boundaries.

BEHAVIOR ENACTMENT IN ACTION

In clinical practice it is not at all uncommon for the therapeutic process to become bogged down, particularly as clients attempt to grapple with highly emotional aspects of their lives. In short-term treatment, where the pressures of time are continually present, therapist and client need ways of surmounting such barriers, and enactment can offer such a tool.

Following the break-up of her marriage, a forty-year-old woman sought help with a pervasive and lingering depression. Conventional exploration of feelings and task assignments aimed at restoring social contact and functioning were only minimally helpful.

As the helping process seemed at an impasse, she was asked to visualize herself in an imaginary dialogue with her ex-husband in which she could talk to him in any manner that might be helpful to her.

In a faltering, hesitant voice she began to speak to him of her anger and hurt about the divorce but stopped, after a few phrases, visibly trembling. Several repetitions of this scene clearly demonstrated, to both her and the therapist, the intensity of her feelings of loss and, most importantly, how frightened she was to express these feelings, even in an imagined encounter.

The powerful, self-directed emotion dislodged even in an apparent simulation became a central theme in subsequent working through of her grief.

There are many helping situations where behavioral enactment can give both therapist and client an opportunity to discover the presence of behavioral or skill deficits. Such gaps in social facility can be easily obscured in purely verbal description, which frequently emphasizes the client's emotional reaction to life events instead of accurately portraying the literal interaction.

For example, a nineteen-year-old part-time college student described a series of failures in obtaining dates with girls and saw much of his dissatisfaction with himself as related to these difficulties. Enactments of his approach to beginning a casual conversation with a young woman—far short, of course, of his goal of dating—revealed extreme difficulty with such basic behaviors as eye contact and initial small talk, and the need for intensive social skill training became apparent.

In other instances it may be that the client's facility with language is simply not sufficient to capture the subleties of tone, gesture, or stance that can significantly qualify social relationships. Enactment allows the client to demonstrate aspects of self that words alone could not convey.

Similarly, behavior that has become repetitive or habitual may be omitted from any verbal description, not as the result of a deliberate act of censorship, but because of its very everydayness—its practiced familiarity. In such cases the behavior enactment, in a deliberate act of simplification, seeks to reveal the importance of the mundane.

In a like vein, the therapist can utilize a behavioral demonstration to portray alternative approaches to an apparent dilemma or to illustrate elements of selected social skills, with an economy and impact far superior to ordinary suggestion and advice. The client then can imitate such demonstrations, receiving necessary guidance and encouragement in an immediate way that pushes beyond the confines of language.

Both therapist and client may be reluctant to utilize this unfamiliar dimension of change. We are most comfortable with conversation, and there is no doubt that the acquisition of language, the ability to express oneself through words, represents one of the most distinctive milestones of human development. Yet Hamlet, in a bright moment of candor disguised as madness, denounced it all as "words, words, words," and from time to time therapists also have become disenchanted with this medium of human interchange. Behavior enactments, in their varied forms, offer an alternative.

Phases of Behavioral Enactment

Behavior enactment and rehearsal methods constitute a readily available means of bridging the gap between words and action yet involve an approach that can be adapted to a wide range of therapeutic orientations and styles without radically altering their character. The major requirement in utilizing this approach is that the helper must be comfortable in entering a visual and physical dimension and, further, must be able to prepare the client for this same transition.

The process of behavior enactment can be conceptualized as containing three potential phases, and the therapist may utilize one or all of these phases. In the first phase, the *enactment* proper, the client is asked to portray how a specific problematic situation is presently managed. In the second phase, *modeling*, the therapist demonstrates an alternative method of coping with the same situation. Finally, in the third phase, *practice* (or rehearsal), the client attempts the same situation again but endeavors to incorporate aspects of the therapist's prior demonstration. After each phase the clinician and client discuss the impact of the enactment, and wherever the client has attempted new responses, the helper must offer consistent reinforcement, assessment, and feedback on these efforts. Similarly, the client must be encouraged to realistically evaluate her or his own level of performance.

In each of the phases, of course, the client and the therapist role-play, or simulate, the participants in the selected situation. Both therapist and client may find that moving into this new dimension can initially evoke considerable discomfort and awkwardness. There is also an implicit challenge in asking people to demonstrate their actions. ''Show me'' has a much more confrontive quality than ''Tell me,'' and therapists often are wary of confrontation, even in minor forms. Similarly, troubled clients may prefer to create a fabric of words around their concerns rather than expose themselves to the uncertain risks of portrayal.

Goldfried and Davison (1976) discuss behavior rehearsal in

their book *Clinical Behavior Therapy* and offer many useful suggestions on its application. They especially emphasize the need to prepare the client for behavioral rehearsal and identify three major therapeutic tasks during this transition:

1. *Client acceptance of the need to develop new behaviors.* Goldfried and Davison (1976) point out that "even though it may be fairly clear that the client's problems stem from a deficiency in certain social skills, the client himself may not be construing his difficulties along these lines" (p, 139). Clients, for example, may see the attitudes or behaviors of others as the sole cause of their difficulties or may ascribe their problems to bad luck or fate. In such extreme instances no therapeutic approach has much chance of success. Fortunately, many clients tend to be uneasily balanced between these unworkable polarities.

Meichenbaum (1975) has similarly stressed the need for client and helper to develop a "common conceptualization" of the goals of therapeutic intervention. In the active context of brief treatment, the therapist must be able to provide clients with a sufficiently hopeful rationale for even attempting to change themselves. Much of the engagement process during the initial interview is aimed at directly eliciting this sort of motivation and shared viewpoint.

2. *Explaining the relevance of behavior rehearsal.* Although clients may accept the position that new responses must be developed, they may have little notion how this can be done. Goldfried and Davison (1976) suggest that the helper begin by explaining behavior rehearsal in rather general outline, providing more specific detail only when it is apparent that the client is interested in attempting the approach. They offer a transcript of a clinical interview (pp. 139–141) which merits close scutiny as the practitioner, through careful redefinition of the client's initial viewpoint and clear explanation of rehearsal procedures, builds a persuasive case for utilizing enactment. This does not mean that one has to be excessively cautious in introducing behavior rehearsal, but the tendency to oversell the approach should be avoided. The practitioner who advocates enactment at the first hint of a

behavioral deficit is more likely to stir up client resistance than to elicit cooperation.

3. *Allaying client awkwardness about behavior enactment.* Finally, Goldfried and Davison (1976) note that "some clients react negatively to behavior rehearsal when it is described to them, partly because they feel this technique would not help them *really* change, and partly because they feel generally awkward about playacting" (p. 139). They suggest that the gradual introduction of enactment procedures helps to diminish this sense of apprehension. On the other hand, I have often found it helpful to manage the client's potential uneasiness by recognizing this uneasiness in the preliminary explanation. Rather than wait for the client to express uncertainty or discomfort, the therapist can incorporate this in his structuring—"You'll find some of this awkward and artificial as we begin, but that will improve as you become more comfortable with the process." In other words, the client's discomfort is redefined as normal and understandable even before it is mentioned, but the possibility of moving beyond this shaky beginning is confidently predicted.

There are many variations possible in employing behavior enactment. Issues in timing, combining, and managing each phase of it will be discussed and illustrated throughout this chapter. Like any helping intervention, behavior enactment must be applied with sensitivity to the unique characteristics and situation of each client. I will discuss each of the phases of behavior enactment in some detail, attempting to identify the essential characteristics of each. Clinical examples will be utilized at a number of points to illustrate the way in which enactment can be introduced to the client, operationalized in different areas of helping practice, and connected to the goal of positive therapeutic change.

THE ENACTMENT PHASE

Therapists are all too familiar with the client who repeatedly describes difficult, even devastating encounters occurring in daily life but appears to have little notion of how to move beyond this level of discourse. Other clients are vague or inarticulate about the problems they are experiencing with family, friends, or associates beyond conveying that these relationships are dissatisfying or frustrating. In other instances, clients may appear to be highly perceptive about the beliefs or emotions that are impeding their reponse, yet this apparent awareness does little to affect change. Something vital is missing, and helper and client alike have become trapped within the limitations of language.

In each of these instances the helping process is effectively stalled. The therapist may have a number of hypotheses about what is affecting the client's ability to cope with the problematic issue, but any efforts to determine such factors will be blunted by the paucity of description offered and the inability of conversation, in its conventional verbal form, to convey the essential elements at play in human relationships. An example from practice will illustrate:

Mrs. Franz saw herself as trapped, after more than twenty years of marriage, in a relationship with a husband whom she perceived as distant and unemotional. She saw him as consistently blocking all her attempts, to improve the relationship and also deal with many concrete matters connected with the daily management of the household and the children. With considerable bitterness she described how impossible it had been, over many years, to obtain his agreement to renovate and redecorate their living room, despite adequate financial ability to do so. The frustration and futility of any effort in this specific area symbolized to her the essential—and unchangeable—stinginess and lack of caring of her husband.

At a descriptive level the impasse was considerable: as long as Mrs. Franz perceived her husband in this light, there was little reason for her to believe that anything other than bitterness and frustration could transpire between them. This, of course, was further compounded by the refusal of Mr. Franz to involve himself in counseling, implicitly confirming his wife's view of his obstinate and ungiving nature. Practically speaking, this also deprived the therapist of any opportunity to directly observe and intervene in their relationship.

It is at a point such as this—a seemingly unsolvable dilemma—that a shift into behavior enactment can be particularly illuminating. Asking Mrs. Franz to demonstrate, within the confines of a simulated role-play with the therapist, how she might initiate a discussion with her husband about redecorating the living room transformed the situation from one of apparent hopelessness into a very different dimension. New possibilities quickly became evident.

Like many clients, Mrs. Franz was reluctant and awkward about actually demonstrating her approach to her husband. After some mild insistence by the therapist and explanation of how the enactment might offer important clues, she attempted the vignette. Several repetitions of the scene were needed before Mrs. Franz could agree that she (and the therapist in the role of husband) were enacting a typical version of the situation.

Almost immediately apparent in the enactment was the profoundly negative manner in which Mrs. Franz approached her husband. Her tone of voice, bodily posture, and gestures all conveyed that she expected refusal and indeed was anxious to get the matter over with, whatever the outcome, as quickly as possible. The verbal content of her request was also negatively phrased—"I don't suppose you want to do anything about the living room?"—and she gave up her effort almost immediately in response to the slightest indication of her husband's disinterest.

Playing the part of the husband, the therapist was struck by the sense of power that he experienced in relation to Mrs. Franz as he noted how easy it was to fend her off, with hardly more than a shrug of indifference.

This brief example illustrates how the helping process must penetrate beyond the conventional in a meaningful way if movement is to occur. Human experience takes place in several dimensions, each of which, alone or in interaction, is capable of assuming prepotency in determining an individual's life choices. Beliefs can become fixed or, as Albert Ellis (1962) has argued, can assume irrational proportions—effectively blocking action or arousing inhibiting affect. Emotions, however aroused, can also pervade our being, with crippling impact upon many aspects of functioning. Finally, the behavioral repertoire itself may be limited, either through a lack of requisite learning or through the habituating effect of repeated interactions, and consequently may offer the individual little sense of self-efficacy (Bandura, 1977a, 1977b) or any realistic opportunity for mastery (Liberman, 1978).

In order to move into behavior enactment, an identifiable interpersonal situation must be isolated that is problematic in some way for the client. The difficulties may be idiosyncratic to a particular relationship. Mrs. Franz was adequately functional in other relationships, and enactments therefore, concentrated on her difficulties in the marital system.

On the other hand, the identified problem may be representative of a wider class of situations in which the client experiences discomfort or conflict. An initial behavior enactment may be a prelude to the extensive employment of this process of therapeutic change, as in assertion or communication training (Lange and Jakubowski, 1976; Wells and Figurel, 1979).

With some clients only the enactment phase will be utilized and the observations that can be made from this sequence will be sufficient to stimulate awareness of facets of approach or response, within the target relationship, that need to be altered. Discussion of alternative approaches, followed by pertinent task assignment, can then take place.

It can sometimes be helpful to audio or videotape the enactment dialogue and replay it with the client in order to facilitate observation and discussion. I have seldom used such equipment in my own practice and find that if the dialogue is kept sufficiently short—two or three minutes is usually enough—accurate recall of the content and relevant cognitions and feelings is possible. Taped reviews of behavior enactments can become too complex, bogged down in detail, and thus risk losing the essential action emphasis of enactment.

Following an enactment there is an opportunity to discuss the behaviors that have been demonstrated or to explore the particular reactions—affective or cognitive—that the client experienced during the vignette. Where the major objective of treatment is to enhance interpersonal or social skills, it is often useful for the therapist to begin the discussion by summarizing major aspects of the role-play. If the client has experienced considerable difficulty in the dialogue, or where the enactment is the first of a gradated series of rehearsals (as, for example, in assertion training), the summary should be carefully selective. It should initially emphasize some *positive* aspect of the client's behavior, however minor, and then point out a very few aspects of the dialogue where specific difficulties were evident.

Lange and Jakuboski's (1976, pp. 155–165) discussion of behavioral rehearsal clearly illustrates the consistent use of this sequence of reinforcement and feedback. Following each enactment (in their case in a group setting) the client is first given encouragement for competent responses and then provided with specific suggestions or modeling for improving skill. Additionally, the client is taught to realistically assess his or her own performance after each vignette. The pacing of learning is critical, and the helper must always be sensitive to the possibility that the enactment itself can become yet another instance of failure, with the client feeling humiliated by the all too obvious deficits protrayed.

The enactment by Mrs. Franz, described earlier, was a typical instance of an intial rehearsal where there was seemingly little of a truly positive nature for the therapist to identify. The helper was hard put to find some glimmer of hopefulness to recognize and, with a considerable effort, suggested to Mrs. Franz, "It must have taken some real courage to even try that situation again, you've been through it so often with such discouraging results." In work with clients attempting to develop social skills, where beginning efforts frequently show little or no real facility, the clinician has to make this same sort of supportive leap.

It is critical, I find, for the therapist to sharply distinguish between enactments that are a prelude to direct behavior change (usually some variant of social skill training) and enactments intended to arouse awareness of conflicted feeling or identify troublesome cognitions. In the latter situations the helper may be much less supportive and indeed may allow the impact of emotion or the recognition of dismaying beliefs and attitudes to build, deliberately inducing stress in the helping encounter. Wachtel (1977), for example, describes enactments with clients experiencing difficulties in close relationships where the deliberate repetition of enactments was needed in order to force the client to face the blocked or evaded emotion.

If the therapist suspects that there are cognitive factors impeding the client's behavior in a particular relationship, it can be helpful to cue the client to look for these as the enactment takes place. "What do you say to yourself as you ask a girl for a date?" stimulated one young man to capture the catastrophic consequences—a slap in the face, or a stinging verbal rejection—that he inwardly anticipated. Despite its name, behavior rehearsal can never be completely behavioral. The skilled therapist maintains a careful balance between the performance aspects of the enactment and the important beliefs, attitudes, and emotions that may be interacting with client behavior. Yet behavior enactment, through bypassing the limitations of descriptive language, offers an opportunity for any (or all) of these elements to be brought into view.

THE MODELING PHASE

After the enactment phase has been discussed and its particular difficulties identified, it is often appropriate for the therapist to demonstrate, in a further simulation, a way in which the situation might be differently handled. In this sequence the helper will assume the part of the client and the client will, of course, play the significant other. Usually the preceding enactment has set the stage sufficiently that the therapist need only briefly describe the reversal of roles and the dialogue can then proceed. Occasionally a client may be reluctant or self-conscious about portraying the other person—whether spouse, employer, or friend—and the therapist will need to encourage the attempt. Acknowledging that the client may feel awkward or foolish in the assumed role is usually sufficient. Most clients are much more anxious about portraying themselves in the enactment phase. This is the far riskier exposure of self, and it is uncommon for any significant reluctance to develop at the modeling phase. Indeed, at times seemingly inhibited clients can play an aggressive spouse or employer with surprising flair and realism.

A critical facet of the modeling phase lies in the selection of exactly what new behaviors to demonstrate. The therapist has to be careful to choose only a very few aspects of new behavior for emphasis and to ensure that these are clearly and unambiguously demonstrated. Such a selection is based, in part, on the difficulties that were evidenced in the prior enactment and pinpointed in the discussion of that phase. In addition, the helper exercises judgment in choosing the elements of more functional behavior that are most likely to be successfully managed by the client in the subsequent rehearsal.

Among a variety of interpersonal problems confronting her, thirty-year-old Joyce B. had emphasized her continuing difficulty in approaching her employer about a potential promotion and salary raise. In an enactment of this dilemma several features of her approach to the employer had stood out: her diffident and meek posture and voice; her reluctance to directly state her concern about the promotion; and finally, a futile reliance on indirect hints about the matter. All of these, in conjunction with a busy, rather insensitive employer, resulted in inevitable failure and further discouragement for Joyce.

In discussing the enactment, the most salient difficulties—her anxious manner and the indirect approach—had been readily identified as problematic, although Joyce, like many clients, was pessimistic about whether she could ever behave any differently.

In the first modeling phase the therapist decided to simplify these difficulties even further: the demonstration concentrated on showing Joyce how some direct eye contact and the essential

phrase "I'd like to talk to you about a promotion" could trans-
form the situation. More subtle aspects of the skills needed to
manage this anxiety-provoking interaction were disregarded and
left for later modeling demonstrations and rehearsals. It was
enough that the client be presented with a very few changes that
she could fairly successfully imitate before attempting to grasp
the totality of the assertive skills involved. As the previous discussion has emphasized, behavioral enactment is an occasion for
learning and growth, not for more challenge and failure. The
helper has to exercise judgment in estimating the boundaries
within which the client can operate, even within the protected
atmosphere of the helping session. The methodology of enactment can give the therapist a handy guideline for intervention, but
as this example illustrates such procedures have to be carefully
guided by the judgment of the skilled helper.

Therapists need to gain facility in utilizing behavior enactment
in much the same way as clients—by actually practicing the
procedures and skills involved. Supervisors, moreover, should
not assume that the inexperienced practitioner, no matter how
familiar with the technical procedures of enactment, is able to
clearly demonstrate social relationship skills. Clinicians planning
to use behavior enactment need to literally practice these skills in
training workshops, supervisory conferences, or with colleagues
in order to gain confidence and facility. The more experienced
practitioner may find it useful to enact particularly difficult situations with consultants or colleagues. As a valuable by-product of
this practical emphasis on performance, I have found that my
own comfort and facility with such vital human skills as assertiveness and intimate communication has increased, not only professionally but personally. There is no reason, of course, why
therapists should not benefit from the same wisdom and practical
learnings they impart to their clients.

THE PRACTICE PHASE

In this final phase of the enactment sequence the elements
demonstrated by the helper are attempted by the client, with an

emphasis on behavioral mastery, and any troublesome cognitions or affects stirred up by this effort are elicited so as to be available for further examination. The importance or pertinence of these aspects of the practice phase will vary from one client to another, or even from time to time for the same client, and therapist will again need to exercise careful judgment about where to place stress.

The attempt at behavioral mastery of the aspects of interpersonal skill that the helper's demonstration highlighted should not be underemphasized. No matter how adequate the client may appear to be in the context of the helping relationship or from descriptions of self in other encounters, the therapist must remember that a perplexing and troubled facet of the client's life is being isolated and examined. It should not be assumed that the helper's demonstration and the client's agreement that this represents a more functional or desirable coping with the situation are a sufficient examination of the dilemma—the behavior must be attempted by the client.

If the client is able to manage a reasonable facsimile of the elements of the modeling selected for emphasis, then the therapist can provide suitable encouragement and either discuss the sequence or move on to another demonstration. Even if the client's effort is labored and flawed, explicit praise of the attempt must be offered. In this latter situation it may well be necessary for the helper to move back to the modeling phase and repeatedly demonstrate the relevant aspects, with the client gradually gaining mastery.

Where the client is experiencing marked difficuly in managing the repetition, the therapist has to exercise considerable care in determining which aspects of the demonstration to emphasize. It is little use trying to teach someone the words to employ in firmly denying an unreasonable request if, for example, his ability to maintain eye contact is minimal or he can speak only in faint, frightened tones. Enactments would have to concentrate on these nonverbal dimensions of assertiveness, through whatever demonstration and practice is needed, before even attempting to work upon the actual verbal content.

It is equally important to identify any critical beliefs and attitudes that may be impeding the client—that one has no right to stand up for oneself, or that one must be liked by everyone—as these may also require change. Indeed, one of the most significant recent advances in assertion training, as well as in behavioral therapy in general, has been the increasing recognition of this cognitive element (Lange and Jakubowski, 1976). This has encouraged the development of *packages* of intervention designed to influence both behavior and thought.

Chapter 9 will discuss the cognitive therapies in greater depth. At this point it will be sufficient to note that access to important cognitions may vary as behavior enactment progresses. I suggested earlier, in discussing the enactment phase, that the clinician should attempt to elicit the client's immediate thoughts as a vignette is attempted. However, at this beginning point, it is not unusual for little except overall discouragement or hesitancy to be forthcoming. In the practice phase, as the client attempts a more adequate response, a different situation may ensue. That is to say, the very attempt to be assertive, for example, may stimulate inhibiting cognitions in a way in which the previously inadequate responses did not. The therapist thus should not assume that client imitation of suggested responses and behaviors is a simple matter of practice and implementation. Higher levels of response, often completely novel to the client, can generate quite unexpected reactions.

The concept of the logical or emotional hierarchy, discussed in Chapter 3, is also highly pertinent to this issue. The helper should be completely familiar with all of the component elements needed in such essential social skills as assertion, intimate communication, and problem solving and be able to quickly identify those missing from the client's repertoire so as to accurately determine the point in the hierarchy where learning must begin. It must be remembered, moreover, that any hierarchy is simply a rough guideline for the practitioner and may require careful adjustment for a particular client. What may seem to the therapist to be an easy and logical transition from one step to the next may represent an awesome leap to the uneasy client.

Similarly, it may be necessary to gauge clients' emotional reaction to any given level of social interaction in order to scale the demands of enactment to their immediate capacity.

Mr. Quinlan, a twenty-two-year-old auto mechanic, had never successfully held a job in his field. He either was fired or quit after a month or two in a position because of his difficulties in getting along with supervisors, fellow workers, and customers. With a wife and two young children to support, he had become increasingly desperate about his problems.

As counseling began, he had just found a new job and was struggling to cope with its demands. He spoke of being bothered by customers who insisted on talking to him as he worked on their cars, and the therapist asked him to enact this situation. The therapist then demonstrated some polite but firm ways of handling customer inquiries, and Mr. Quinlan attempted to practice these. Midway through the rehearsal he became visibly upset and was unable to manage even a mildly assertive response. Recognizing his anxiety, the therapist moved to much simpler levels of social skill and additionally contracted to teach Mr. Quinlan ways of managing the pervading tensions he was experiencing on the job.

FURTHER CLINICAL APPLICATIONS

In the clinical setting perhaps the predominant use of behavior enactment and rehearsal methods has been to teach the client new ways of coping with specific life situations (Goldfried and Davison, 1976). Many therapists are familiar with the employment of behavioral rehearsal in such structured change procedures as social skill or assertion training. Indeed, the major area of documentation for its effectiveness as a teaching device has been in assertion training (McFall and Lilliesand, 1971; McFall and Twentyman, 1973). It would be a pity, however, if we were to limit usage of this powerful tool to only a narrow range of applications. Enactments can be utilized in many helping situations and adapted to a variety of therapeutic orientations and styles;

their employment need be limited only by the imagination of the therapist and the unique life goals of the client.

Enactments are especially adaptable to very brief contacts where a specific difficuly, often of some urgency to the individual, needs to be dealt with in a focused way. For example, behavior enactment and rehearsal have been utilized in work in a hospital setting with patients who are experiencing anxiety around discussing their medical condition with their physician.* This problem can be aggravated in a large hospital by the impersonality of a busy medical staff, and the patient will often feel extremely frustrated and defeated after repeated but ineffectual attempts to gain information.

Since at least some of the difficulty experienced by such patients may arise from anxiety about their condition, it is usually helpful, prior to any enactment, to spend some time with the individual writing down a list of the questions he would like to ask the physician. This not only concretizes the goal of the intervention—obtaining specific medical information—but also has some effect in moderating the patient's anxiety about these questions as they assume a more tangible form. There is also opportunity during this phase to shape certain of the patient's beliefs—by statements such as "You have a right to this information," "You have to take responsibility to get it," or "You often have to teach your doctor how to talk to you"—so as to prepare for later steps in the intervention.

The therapist makes the transition to behavior enactment, once the basic concern is clearly established, by beginning to question the patient about the specifics of his or her previous encounters with the physician. The form of the questions—"How did you ask the doctor?" "What did you say then?" or "What did the doctor do?"—is designed to make the patient aware of the actual behaviors in the situation and to serve as a natural prelude to behavior enactment. It is best for the therapist to take the initial risk of enacting by explaining that it is still unclear from the

*I am indebted to Larry V. Pacoe, Ph.D., for this illustrative material.

verbal description what is going wrong and adding that it might be helpful for the therapist to play the part of the doctor so that the patient can convey his or her concerns more clearly. From this initial enactment it is an easy transition to further modeling or practice sequences that will enhance the patient's ability to cope with the encounter.

The essential step, it must be emphasized, is to give the patient some explicit practice in actually stating the specific questions to the physician. The written list that patient and therapist have already worked out is, of course, highly useful, but the actual experience, in enactment, of voicing these concerns cannot be omitted. During the rehearsal it is also possible to teach the patient some simple techniques that will be useful in managing some of the common difficulties that may arise. For example, lightly placing a hand on the physician's arm can stop him from walking away; simply saying "I don't understand" can be a response to unclear medical terminology. The intervention is concluded by instructing the patient to keep the prepared list of questions nearby and to actually use it in the session with the physician. Additionally, the therapist should make a note on the patient's chart to the effect that "the patient has a number of questions." Finally, the therapist should initiate a follow-up interview with the patient in which the meeting with the doctor will be reviewed, gaps in the information obtained will be discussed, and any new questions will be identified and rehearsed.

A more general clincial application can be seen in Lange and Jakubowski's (1976) volume on assertion training, which outlines a sequence for behavior rehearsal that is highly adaptable to many other problematic social and interpersonal situations. Their model emphasizes a series of successive enactments by the client in which the elements of adaptive response to a complex situation are gradually developed in a step-by-step fashion. During this phase of skill enhancement the role of the antagonist (boss, spouse, peer, etc.) is carefully controlled so as to avoid any reactions that might be unmanageable for the learner during the early stages of development. Each enactment in the series concentrates upon a few clearly defined (or modeled) aspects of the desired behavior, and following each rehearsal the client is given immediate encouragement and feedback.

Only after the client has gained reasonable facility and confidence in coping with the situation are more difficult or conflictful elements introduced into the antagonist's role. Lange and Jakubowski (1976) describe this approach in relation to a young woman attempting to deal with a difficult employer:

> Judy then practiced several more interactions. At first the employer was encouraged to be cooperative and support the request. When Judy successfully completed the entire scene to her satisfaction, the trainer then asked her to practice the scene with the employer responding negatively (e.g., anger, threat, indifference, guilt, or whatever "hooks" her). The situation was then practiced until *Judy was satisfied* with how she assertively handled the employer's uncooperative response. [pp. 161-162].

In effect this is yet another illustration of the learning hierarchy and can be seen as a combination of the logical (simple to complex) and the emotional (least anxious to most anxious) elements of this learning paradigm. In addition, this adaptation of the behavior enactment model draws upon an aspect of the approach that has considerable clinical significance—*behavior rehearsal is simultaneously real and unreal.* Although enactments are capable of arousing very tangible emotions or revealing significant skill deficits, they are *not* the real-life situation. The imaginative therapist can capitalize on this characteristic of enactment to protect the client, particularly during the early stages of change, and thus heighten the possibility of effective learning.

Finally, Lange and Jakubowski (1976) discuss the combination of relaxation training with behavior rehearsal procedures. No matter how much the clinician may simplify the rehearsal situation, there are some clients who become quite anxious at even elementary levels of enactment. Mr. Quinlan, the harried auto mechanic described earlier in this chapter, was an obvious example of this sort of person. Teaching the client some simple tension reduction methods—relaxing words, calming scenes, deep breathing—may be necessary in order to make participation possible. Even for those who do not appear to be unduly tense, the acquisition of stress management techniques can be a highly useful adjunct to the behavioral and cognitive changes induced through behavior rehearsal. Chapter 8 of this book will discuss stress management approaches in greater detail.

These few examples, will convey some notion of the adaptability of enactment procedures to various situational contexts and diverse client characteristics. In subsequent chapters further uses of behavior enactment methods will be considered. Their value will be especially evident as the development of social skills is reviewed. Modeling and rehearsal procedures are heavily utilized within the therapeutic interview to assist the individual in skill development. Similarly, cognitive changes in a number of key areas are often identified and induced through variations on enactment.

Chapter 7

Tasks and Homework

One must put tasks in their way which they can accomplish and from the accomplishment of which they gain faith in themselves.
—Alfred Adler

The concept of a task as a means of controlling or shaping one's destiny has played an integral part in human endeavour throughout history.* Such heroes of mythology and folklore as Hercules were required to demonstrate their worthiness and courage through seemingly impossible task accomplishment. The miller's daughter in *Rumpelstiltskin*, to her utter dismay, found she had to prove her suitability for marriage to the king by weaving straw into gold. At an everyday level, we all know the satisfaction of completing a piece of work, obtaining an excellent grade in a course, or mastering a new facet of a sport or hobby. Whether heroic or ordinary, the task confronts us with challenge from the environment and with an opportunity to demonstrate our capacity to cope with the demands of living.

The use of tasks has become particularly developed and refined in short-term treatment, and this chapter will review certain key aspects of such theory and practice. Initially, however, I will survey the history of task usage across all psychotherapeutic approaches. Liberman's (1978) discussion of the concept of mas-

---

*The assistance of two former students, Rosemary Armany and Barbara Lonardi, in gathering material on which parts of this chapter are based is gratefully acknowledged.

tery will be utilized as a central theoretical construct underlying task assignment, and a number of secondary factors will be related to this core theme. A classification of tasks as observational, experiential, or incremental will be suggested, and clinical examples will be employed to illustrate these categories. Finally, methods of improving task performance and dealing with common difficulties in clinical application will be dicussed.

Tasks in Clinical Practice: A Brief History

In one of the few intensive discussions of the employment of tasks and homework in therapeutic practice, Shelton and Ackerman (1974) define tasks as "assignments given to the client which are carried on outside the therapy hour" (p. 3). While many therapists may employ tasks on an irregular basis, a major characteristic of planned short-term treatment is to utilize homework in a consistent, systematic manner throughout the intervention.

Precedent for the use of assignments to be completed outside the therapy session is not difficult to find. Dunlap (1932), for example, contended that clients could learn to extinguish unwanted behaviors through the use of repeated homework assignments. An early work by Herzberg (1941) offered a similar rationale. Salter (1949) described patients with a wide range of difficulties utilizing self-instigation to effect changes in their own behavior. Stevenson (1959) underscored the importance of homework in enhancing the development of assertive, affiliative, and communication skills.

While more recent writers have mentioned homework assignments, they have generally relegated tasks to occasional use in, for instance, dealing with isolated aspects of client difficulty. These include such authors as Bach and Wyden (1968), Storrow (1967), and Wolpe and Lazarus (1966). Only Haley (1976), among the nonbehavioral writers, has examined the employment of tasks with any degree of sophistication, and I will consider certain of his ideas later in this chapter.

A recent review by Shelton (1979) identifies three major influences underlying the development of therapeutic homework. The first of these, as Chapter 3 noted, is the notion of instigative therapy, particularly as conceptualized by Kanfer (1979). In this view of the therapeutic process, emphasis is placed on change taking place *outside* of the actual therapy session. The interview situation is seen as an opportunity to plan how such change will be initiated and to systematically review the client's attempts to achieve this. The instigative perspective is heavily dependent, of course, on a means to carry out such attempts, and the development of realistic and flexible task assignments becomes a necessary ingredient of the approach.

A second major influence, as Shelton points out, has been the direct sex therapy approaches pioneered by Masters and Johnson (1970), which were among the first to employ systematic homework assignments as an integral aspect of the therapy. Moreover there is evidence that task compliance is essential to effective sex therapy. For example, Lansky and Davenport (1975) describe a relatively unsuccessful series of sexual therapy cases but at the same time report that most of their clients did not carry out the prescribed homework. Lanasky and Davenport point out an almost exact correspondence between those clients who carried out the exercises and those who benefited from treatment.

Finally, Shelton's own work has been a factor in promoting the planned use of tasks and assignments, and his monograph on the utilization of homework in psychotherapy (Shelton and Ackerman, 1974) is certainly a significant contribution. In addition, Shelton has been active in the empirical examination of the effects of task assignment and in several studies (Shelton, 1973, 1975; Chesney and Shelton, 1976) has demonstrated its positive effects in enhancing change.

FURTHER INFLUENCES

Two further sources of influence on task utilization need to be recognized. Within the social work field the efforts of William

Reid in the development of task-centered casework have been especially significant. Thus Reid and Epstein (1972) point out that their development of task-centered casework was stimulated by the notion of drawing upon the "natural task-setting and task-achieving of individuals in difficulty" (p. 94–95). Reid and his colleagues not only have pioneered an approach which places explicit emphasis upon task accomplishment but have persistently gathered empirical data supporting various facets of the method. Reid's work on the "Task Implementation Sequence" (1975)—a procedure for enhancing the probability that the client will undertake assigned homework—will be examined in greater detail later in this chapter.

Additionally, the employment of tasks and directives within the field of family therapy has many implications for short-term therapy generally. A number of family therapists who might not consider themselves short-term therapist have utilized tasks extensively, both in and out of the therapeutic session. Salvador Minuchin (1974, 1978), in some of his most recent explications of structural family therapy, offers many examples of this approach.

There are two major ways in which Minuchin and other family therapists have employed tasks. First, there are instances where the structural family therapist will ask a family member to try out a new bit of behavior right in the therapeutic session. Thus a husband may be instructed to help his wife talk to their teen-age son about a difficult topic. In another family the task might be for the father to do exactly the opposite—to allow his wife to talk to their son without in any way participating. In an initial interview, contained in his volume on work with anorexia nervosa, Minuchin (Minuchin et al., 1978) asks for a shift in the family's seating arrangement in order to challenge their habitual patterns of interaction:

> *Minuchin:* Can you answer your mother, Loretta? Carlo, let Mama sit near Loretta. Loretta, talk with Mother, because she says that you are controlling the house [p. 307].

In all of these examples the therapist is suggesting certain behaviors for the client and the task is to try them out immediately. This use of tasks within the therapeutic session is obviously quite similar to the enactment methods discussed in Chapter 6.

Minuchin also discusses the use of tasks in a manner analogous to the instigative approach—that is to say, as activities to be carried out *between* therapy sessions. In the same initial interview cited above Minuchin concludes the session by asking the father and daughter to spend at least half an hour twice during the following week talking together about themselves. His instructions are very explicit:

> *Minuchin:* For this week, before you return again, I want you, Loretta, to talk to your father twice for half an hour. Carlo, you will select two evenings to talk with your daughter. Today is what? Friday? Talk with him during the weekend one time and talk with him next week, Loretta. If she doesn't do that, you make the time, Carlo, and you say, ''I want you to know me,'' and you talk no more than half an hour.
> *Father:* Okay.
> *Minuchin:* No more than half an hour and twice during this week, Loretta... [Minuchin et al., 1978, p. 322]

Minuchin's approach to giving task assignments is exemplary, offering a clear model for this aspect of the therapeutic art. The reader should note carefully for example, how directly and succinctly the task is prescribed. There is no doubt about what Minuchin is asking of his clients, and his vocabulary is simple and entirely nontechnical. He describes when, where, and how the task is to be carried out and furthermore keeps its demands extremely limited. It is difficult for the family members to complain that talking together twice for half an hour each time is too burdensome an assignment.

TASKS AND MASTERY

Liberman (1978) suggests that successful task accoplishment promotes ''a feeling of mastery, control over one's internal reactions and relevant external events'' (p. 75) and consequently plays an indispensable role in maintaining individual self-esteem. His analysis of the role of mastery, both in daily living and as an effective ingredient in psychotherapy, is highly pertinent to the consideration of tasks that is the subject of this chapter. Much of the following discussion is heavily indebted to Liberman's review.

He points out that many different psychotherapies have directly or indirectly utilized the concept of mastery. For some therapies task performance will take place within the actual therapeutic session and may consist, for instance, in recalling dreams, exploring feelings, or actively participating in emotionally arousing procedures. For other therapies the emphasis is on task assignment outside of the session and the client will be directed to visit with extended family members, practice relaxation exercises, read selected books and articles, and so on. The commonality of these many approaches to task performance may lie, not in the physical location or the specific nature of the task activity, but in its requirement by the therapist as a socially sanctioned expert. Implicit in this requirement is the belief conveyed to the client that following such procedures will lead to relief from suffering.

However, whether task performance will promote mastery depends upon the manner in which the person approaches and interprets his or her performance. Liberman reviews a series of research studies which identify five factors that can significantly influence this interpretation. In sum, these factors can be regarded as a conceptual framework within which the client is likely to view the assigned task:

Background variables. There appear to be individuals whose personal background and current environment make them especially open to change efforts. Some of the research findings confirm the not surprising conclusion that, on the average, such factors as middle-class background, college education, and white-collar occupation tend to support the impetus toward mastery. In contrast, people from working-class, low socioeconomic, or ghetto backgrounds are more likely to see their lives as externally controlled and, as Liberman emphasizes, "primarily a matter of luck, fate, chance or some powerful outside agent" (p. 41). Hence clients from these latter groups will more often request help with concrete aspects of their environment or immediate context of living.

However, both empirically and clinically the matter is not as simple as one of middle-class people necessarily being the most "desirable" clients. The more intellectually inclined client, for example, may stay at this level, hesitating to put his or her verbal awareness into any concrete form. On the other hand, Burgoyne and his colleagues (1979), as I pointed out in Chapter 5, found that lower socioeconomic clients often desire the more specifically therapeutic forms of helping but tend to *combine* this request with requests of a more tangible nature. Difficulties arise when the therapist, biased perhaps by the common clinical beliefs about the low socioeconomic group, responds only to the concrete request. Tasks can serve as a middle ground between these two polarities, offering a means of testing out insights in action or, with the more practically oriented client, providing a vehicle for developing greater emotional or cognitive awareness.

Task relevance. As Liberman emphasizes, "a person's involvement and commitment to a task are also dependent upon the relevance of the task for him" (p. 43). Any psychotherapy can be viewed as containing a series of tasks even if these are not conducted outside of the session, but clients must see these tasks as meaningfully related to solving the difficulties they are experiencing. Free association or interpretation in analytically oriented therapy or the relaxation procedures of systematic desensitization, from this viewpoint, will not have optimal effect unless the client views them as pertinent to problem resolution. The same considerations apply to tasks carried out in the natural environment.

Two major implications for practice can be drawn from this construct:

1. Difficulty around task relevance can be avoided if the helper utilizes homework assignments that are directly related to

the goals of change desired by the client. This may appear to be an obvious consideration, yet many practitioners hesitate to work directly upon the client's difficulties in living. It may seem almost embarrassingly simplistic to suggest to the client that problems in close relationships, for example, can be improved through deliberately increasing one's personal contacts or that leaving the parental home can involve little more than planning and carrying out the steps needed in making such a move. Too often our theories have suggested that the solutions to all problems *must* be complex and indirect, and consequently clinicians have lost the ability to be simple and immediate.

2. The client's understanding of the relevance of a task can be heightened by adequate explanation from the therapist. The theories that undergird therapeutic intervention are essentially explanations of the process of change and, suitably conveyed to the client, can serve a highly useful purpose in explaining such treatment procedures as task assignment. Many of the concepts of clinical theory, for better or worse, have become incorporated into the common knowledge of North American society. For example, the emphasis of ego psychology on defense mechanisms and social learning theory's identification of habit formation and skill deficits are familiar concepts to many clients. This does not mean that the practitioner should indulge in lengthy jargon-filled lectures, but it does suggest that suitable explanation can serve a vital purpose in enhancing task relevance. Additionally, the clinician's comprehensive grasp of theory can assist in varying such explanation to the needs of the poorly educated client, as well as to those of higher educational levels.

Task difficulty. The experience of mastery gained from performing a task is also related to the perceived difficulty of the assignment. For instance, as Liberman points out, "tasks which are perceived as too easy to too difficult yield feelings neither of success nor of failure" (p. 45). On the other hand, though certain tasks may be so complex that the behaviors necessary for their performance are not within the client's existing repertoire, there are instances where even unsuccessfully attempting a very difficult task can significantly bolster the individual's ability to cope with less demanding tasks in the same problem area.

All of these considerations suggest that the clinician must exercise some care in task selection. The task must in general be one that the individual is able to carry out, yet demanding enough that its performance has meaning. Some clinicians suggest that the task should represent a distinctly higher level than the client's present functioning. For example, in their discussion of tasks in rational-emotive therapy Walen and her colleagues (1980) suggest that "large steps" be employed in order to challenge the client. This is reminiscent, of course, of the approach utilized in the implosive or emotional flooding approaches (Stampfl and Levis, 1867), where the client, in imagery or *in vivo,* is confronted with the most demanding situations possible. Most clinicians, however, prefer to follow the principles of shaping and, except in unusual circumstances, choose task assignments at the simpler and less anxiety-provoking end of the client's subjective continuum. Certainly the employment of shaping methods has the firmest empirical substantiation and should be utilized in most cases. But the clinician should not be *excessively* cautious, and judgment must be exercised to ensure that the task is not too simple or nondemanding.

Attitudes of significant others. The manner in which important people in the client's life react to a task may affect the meaningfulness of the performance. Despite the client's initial trepidations, many of the significant people in the immediate environment will be surprisingly supportive of change. Some theories to the contrary, we should not regard the natural environment (or the people that populate it) as necessarily malevolent or inherently unhelpful. To the contrary, there is more reason to see the natural remedial forces as at least as helpful as anything we can offer within the therapeutic arena, and as I have frequently emphasized, the effective therapist makes every effort to tap this resource.

At the same time, Liberman suggests that the therapist, during the course of treatment, often assumes the role of a significant ɔther and can play an influential part in supporting task performance:

> The therapist can heighten the effects of success by praise and approval and can ameliorate the effects of failure by indicating that the poor performance has not diminished his request for the patient [p. 46].

Liberman notes that a task may be carried out, at least in the early stages of treatment, in order to please the therapist, but like most short-term practitioners, he regards this as acceptable motivation at this beginning point. His emphasis on the importance of therapist attitude toward task performance also underscores the necessity of the therapist's following up on task assignment. If the clinician neglects to inquire about the client's performance on an assigned task, an attitude of depreciation may be implicitly conveyed and the client will invest less in future tasks.

Attribution of performance. Finally, it is essential that the individual believe that performance on a task is the result of his own efforts and that success or failure can be ascribed to himself. If the client sees his efforts as due to luck or fate or to the intervention of others, then his own role will be significantly diminished or, in some cases, entirely disqualified. The therapist must look for opportunities to influence the client's attribution processes so as to heighten the probability of self-attribution. Liberman suggests certain tactics:

> The therapist can also play a role in the attribution process by convincing the patient that his gains are due to the patient's own efforts. . . . Conversely the therapist can reattribute failures so that the patient does not view them as presumed defects in character [p. 46].

The importance of the clinician's carefully monitoring client attribution as tasks are carried out cannot be overemphasized. It is deflating, to say the least, to discover, *after* a series of tasks have been performed, that the client has ascribed his success to pure luck or, worse still, entirely to the therapist's support and guidance. On the other hand, as difficult a situation can develop if the client has failed at a task and attributes this entirely to his own inadequacy or incompetence. Perhaps not surprisingly, clients seldom blame the practitioner for task failure ("If you hadn't told me to do it. . . ''), although this is a common apprehension of beginning therapists. I will discuss some further methods of redirecting attributions in a later section of this chapter.

A Task Classification

Tasks have been categorized in a variety of ways. Reid (1975), for example, speaks of *unique* tasks which require a one-time performance by the client ("Get information on the child care facilities in your immediate neighborhood") and *repeated* tasks which ask the client to act in a particular way in a series of situations ("Talk briefly to someone in your class every day this week"). Haley (1976) divides tasks into two distinct categories based upon the therapist's intent in task assignment:

> . . . (1) telling people what to do when the therapist wants them to do it, and (2) telling people what to do when the therapist does *not* want them to do it—because the therapist wants them to change by rebelling [p. 52].

Tasks in Haley's second category, also called paradoxical tasks, have been a subject of considerable fascination for many clinicians. Actually there is paradoxical undertone to all task assignment—how else can one ask anxious or depressed clients to carry out some version of the very behaviors they fear and avoid? The *explicitly* paradoxical task, however, will not be discussed in any detail in this book. Instead I will concentrate on the large proportion of tasks utilized in clinical practice that are relatively straightforward in their intent to pinpoint or stimulate change. Within this overall category of tasks three sub-categories can be distinguished.

1. *Observational or monitoring tasks.* These are tasks whose

main purpose is to gather more information on a selected aspect of the client's life or, in other instances, to increase the individual's awareness of significant behaviors, emotions, or beliefs in a given area of difficulty.

2. *Experiential tasks.* There are times when a task is deliberately designed to arouse emotion in the client or to challenge beliefs or attitudes that are playing an integral part in maintaining the individual's problem. This type of task is particularly applicable where passivity or the repetitive use of ineffectual behaviors is maintaining or worsening the difficulties.

3. *Incremental change tasks.* The tasks in this category are designed to stimulate change directly toward a desired goal, in a step-by-step manner. Incremental tasks are usually devised in an interrelated sequence and arranged along a logical or emotional hierarchy relevant to the client's personal style and particular area of difficulty.

OBSERVATIONAL OR MONITORING TASKS

In the beginning phases of brief therapy the therapist will frequently ask clients to keep a log or diary of some selected aspect of their lives. Parents concerned about a child's behavior can be instructed to keep a record of the child's activities with friends. An adult can be asked to keep track of every interpersonal contact over a given week. Another client may be requested to keep a log of the amount of food consumed each day and the circumstances in which eating occurs. The variety of possible observational assignments is limited only by the imagination of the helper and, of course, the specific needs of the client.

In an initial interview with a young man, recently separated from his wife, it was apparent that he was almost deliberately isolating himself from social contacts. Although he verbalized his strong feelings of loneliness, he was narrowing his world to the few people he saw on his job. An early task was to ask him to begin recording, in simple diary form, any human contacts he experienced during his evenings or weekends. It as emphasized that this would help in understanding who was available to him. Additionally, it was hoped that his awareness of the manner in which crisis was constricting him would be dramatized.

This type of assignment is, obviously, borrowed from the behavioral therapists and serves some of the same purposes that they identify. It establishes a baseline of frequency for a problematic behavior and adds further specification to the problem definition already worked out with the client. If the client is concerned about drinking, for example, how often does this occur, and under what circumstances? Where the client wants to develop certain social skills, it is usually necessary to know something more about his or her present level of skill. Like behavioral enactment, tasks add flesh to the verbal descriptions obtained within the interview.

Tasks in which the client follows a particular aspect of life, recording its occurrence and observing its characteristics, are especially useful as treatment begins. It is at this point that more detail is needed. One of the disadvantages of the relatively rapid process of engagement by which short-term treatment is initiated is the lack of such detail. Tasks of this kind, over the first two or three interviews, fill in these gaps. Thus the therapist can often concentrate on relationship development in the initial interview rather than elaborate problem exploration; knowing that such informative devices as behavior enactments and observational assignments are easily mobilized in the early stages of treatment allows such latitude.

This is not to say that the use of diaries or logs should be restricted to the early sessions. One of the major benefits of this type of homework assignment at later stages of therapy lies in the perspective it can offer on the ongoing therapeutic work. Many therapists are familiar, I am sure, with the situation where the client begins to describe a problem that came up during the preceding week. As the description continues, affect is aroused—discouragement or anxiety, let us say—and it becomes exceedingly difficult to disentangle events and emotions. If the client has been assigned to keep a daily diary focused, let us say, on interpersonal contacts, then a very different picture can be seen. From the diary it is possible to ascertain, for example, that one or perhaps two days were difficult, while the others were not. This is very different from having to rely on the client's entirely selective recollection of the week and to find later, as so often happens, that his recollection is highly skewed. Even if the diary reveals that every day contained difficulties, at least this is a more concrete indication of the client's present level of functioning than his or her unaided recollection.

Observational assignments can be shaped to fit the style of the particular client. Some individuals respond very well to a concrete and specific form of recording in which a chart with suitable headings is worked out and the behaviors of interest are appropriately noted. Others are less responsive or even antagonistic to this approach, viewing it as too mechanical or constricting. In such situations the client can be asked to keep a diary, with a much greater literary or poetic license allowed in the recording. The point is that the clients attempt to observe their life activities in a manner that is more systematic and self-conscious than their typical fashion.

In two of the cases described in Chapter 3 daily logs were utilized. Both Mr. Jurecko, in his attempts to gain greater control of his anger, and Mr. Faber, whose concern was to develop increased confidence in relationship to women, kept such charts at points in the treatment process. However, there were some subtle differences in the purpose of each assignment that bear further discussion at this time.

Mr. Jurecko was instructed to record in his notebook any incidents at work that were upsetting to him. He was simply asked to make a brief note of these so that he and the therapist could gain a better notion of the frequency and severity of episodes that were likely to increase his stress level or to provoke anger. The clinician's intent in this assignment was to heighten Mr. Jurecko's awareness of stress-producing incidents and, further, to obtain a somewhat more objective estimate of the effect of the tension reduction methods that Mr. Jurecko was beginning to learn.

The employment of a daily log came at a somewhat different point in intervention with Mr. Faber and consequently had a different purpose. He was not asked to keep a count, so to speak, of discrete episodes, but was to use a particular type of event as a signal for closer examination of himself. Specifically, he was to attempt to become more aware of the thoughts and fantasies— positive or negative—that occurred when he was in close association with a woman. The recording of these observations was to take place at a convenient time after the event and was more in the nature of keeping a personal diary than doing a behavioral or numerical type of charting. The purpose, of course, was to stimulate and uncover any intruding cognitions that were interfering with his ability to manage these relationships.

In a similar vein, the recently developed cognitive restructuring approaches to the treatment of depression and anxiety (Beck, 1976) also employ observational tasks as an integral element in the therapeutic process. Burns and Beck (1978) describe a "Daily Record of Dysfunctional Thoughts" which the client is trained to use:

> This is a form that patients fill out on a daily basis between therapy sessions and record their uncomfortable emotions (including sadness, anxiety or anger) as well as negative thoughts. They are then to write down a rational response to the negative thought and monitor the degree of emotional relief they experience [p. 128].

This task, it will be noted, goes somewhat beyond simple observation as the client not only tracks disturbing thoughts and emotions but attempts to control the negative cognition through substituting a rational response.

There are many advantages in beginning a task at the observational level, even if the therapist is well aware that the task may implicitly involve elements of challenge or change. It is helpful, during the initial assignment of such a task, to place greatest emphasis on its monitoring aspects. That is to say, the information that carrying it out will provide should be stressed. The attempt to alter negative cognitions or to attain emotional relief (as in the example above) should be pictured as strictly experimental and quite likely to be difficult to manage in any consistent way.

By downplaying the more active portion of the assignment at these early stages, the practitioner can reduce much of the pressure concerning success or failure that the client may feel about task performance. This is an especially important consideration in working with individuals who are already placing an inordinate demand upon themselves and whose sense of demoralization is great. In effect, the therapist's effort is to present the task in such a way that it is practically impossible for the client not to achieve some measure of success.

EXPERIENTIAL TASKS

When life difficulties arise that the individual cannot manage, a common human reaction is to wait for circumstances to change so that the problem will resolve itself in some spontaneous manner. At other times the person will repeatedly attempt a previously successful solution in the hope that, sooner or later, the desired results will ensue. There is nothing inherently wrong or irrational in either of these commonsense tactics, but, at an extreme, either may act to compound or perpetuate existing difficulties. Thus the need for action can be inhibited by inaction or passivity; creative response can be blocked by the repetition of familiar but now unworkable responses.

Experiential tasks are designed to help the baffled client break through impasses of this sort. It is not at all surprising, of course, to find that people in difficulty have drastically limited their range of behavior and in many instances are repetitively enacting unworkable patterns of reaction and response. At much less stressful levels parents scold and nag, children belligerently rebel, despondent individuals reduce their association with others, and the more aggressive respond with overt hostility. Hansell (1973, 1975) sees these repetitive patterns as an integral, though dysfunctional, part of the normal human response to accumulated stress or crisis. The experiential task is utilized to stimulate the individual to break our of this habitual pattern or at least to challenge the patterns of emotional arousal and negative thought that maintain it.

Experiential tasks come in many forms. Haley (1976) describes a case in which a eight-year-old boy was seen because of his strong fear of dogs. The fear was having adverse effects on the child's emotional stability and social adjustment, and a year of insight-oriented individual therapy had done little to resolve it. The task-oriented therapist gave an early assignment to the boy and his parents: they were to purchase "a dog that was afraid," and, together, the boy and his family were to help the animal overcome its fears. Whatever else one may conjecture about this task, its experiential elements are clear.

Similarly, the homework tasks categorized by Walen et al. (1980) as *action assignments* have a significant experiential component. These authors combine such tasks with a rational-emotive approach (see Chapter 9) and subdivide them further into risk-taking or shame-attacking variants. In either case the underlying purpose is to challenge clients' fixed beliefs about themselves or the nature of their world.

Risk-taking assignments may call upon the client, for example, actually to have an experience with failure. Thus Walen et al. (1980) describe a young man with dating anxiety who was instructed, not to make three successful social contacts, but to "go out and collect three *rejections* in the next week" (p. 225). Their use of shame-attacking assignments is even more dramatic: "Go up to a stranger and greet him or her warmly. Ask about his or her health. Be effusive" or "Yell out five successive stops in the subway or bus" (p. 226). As they point out, these assignments, aside from arousing strong emotion, are designed to "challenge the dire need for conventionality... and... help clients evaluate the accuracy of their predictions of how the world will react to them" (pp. 226–227).

Experiential tasks are especially applicable in situations where the client is struggling with immobilizing depression or anxiety. Indeed, the cognitive approaches to these widely prevalent mood disorders (Beck, 1976; Burns and Beck, 1978), in addition to restructuring the client's thinking processes (see Chapter 9), place a heavy reliance on tasks designed to provide new experiences to the sufferer. Burns and Beck (1978) succinctly discuss the underlying assumptions of the approach:

> The thoughts, feelings and behaviors of depressed or anxious individuals typically interact in a predictable manner. Because the patient takes his cognitions seriously and places a high degree of belief in his thoughts, he tends to experience many adverse emotions. He then takes these emotions as confirmatory evidence that his beliefs are in fact correct [p. 110].

Unless this self-perpetuating cycle is breached, there is little likelihood of the person's gaining control of the depressive or anxious reaction. Burns and Beck go on to describe a thirty-five-year-old salesman who had been caught up in chronic depression since a divorce six years earlier. As the depression worsened, he found it more and more difficult to maintain his job and began to spend increasing amounts of time at home, ruminating on his difficulties and seriously considering suicide. The therapist directly confronted him with this cyclical pattern of inaction and emotion and assigned him the twofold task of contacting his employer and visiting one customer. Like some experiential tasks the immediate effects were salutory:

> The employer expressed support and empathy and assured him that his job was not in danger. When he called on the customer, he did receive some ribbing about ''being on vacation'' for the past six weeks, but also landed a small order. He later reported with surprise that the discomfort of being teased was actually quite small in comparison with the intense depression he experienced every day at home avoiding work. [pp. 125-126].

Burns and Beck (1978) regard a series of such experiences as necessary to lessen the depressed client's pervasive conviction that he is worthless and inadequate. However, they do not see tasks alone as sufficient and caution the clinician that "the tendency of some depressives to maintain such beliefs despite considerable evidence to the contrary is quite impressive" (p. 120). Indeed, it would be a mistake for the therapist to assume that an experiential task will automatically induce the desired changes. Although some clinical writings suggest that this occurs, such "Eureka!" reactions are relatively rare, and the client more often needs considerable help from the therapist to gain maximum benefit from tasks of any sort. The conceptual framework suggested by Liberman and reviewed earlier in this chapter can be utilized in this process of examining and potentiating task performance.

Thus task relevance should not be viewed as a static client perception, but can be heightened by therapist activity and attitude toward prescribed homework. Relevance is underscored by careful follow-up and review, and the clinician is well advised to inquire about an assigned task at the beginning of the succeeding session with the client—"Let's begin by discussing the assignment you were to work on." Direct inquiry of this kind offers a more specific entry point into the interview than the ubiquitous "How did things go this week?" and additionally tends to promote the focused discussion needed in brief intervention.

The issue of attribution of performance has already been emphasized as critical to task performance and particularly to the development of mastery. However, the clinician may need to approach this facet of client perception rather cautiously, in contrast to the directness employed in other areas of task management. As clients describe or discuss their task performance, the practitioner must listen carefully for indications of attribution and, as the client's viewpoint becomes apparent, consider how this might be handled. The object is to avoid precipitating the client's ascription of attribution prematurely, especially where this may prove problematic. Difficulties can arise in relation to either success or failure: the dispirited client may disclaim any credit for success or, conversely, may entirely embrace failure. The clinician's goal, of course, is to support positive attributions and conversely to decrease negative attributions.

Reinforcement and redefinition, direct or implicit, are the major tactics for influencing attribution. During the client's description of task performance the therapist will look for any opportunity to highlight aspects of the client's reported activities that suggest initiative, courage, determination, creativity, and the like. Sometimes I have had clients report that an assignment went well on one occasion but badly on another. I will then suggest that we talk about the "failure" experience first, explaining to the client that one often learns more from adversity than from success. Implicit in this redefinition is the suggestion that the client has done well even while failing at a task.

In any case, as tasks are performed and change (at whatever level) takes place, the practitioner should exercise great care to ascribe *all* of this success to the efforts of the client. The very direct manner in which this can be done is apparent in an interview transcript reported by Haley (1976). In the same case where the therapist had directed the parents and child to purchase "a dog that was afraid," the therapist later referred back to the successful accomplishment of this task:

> *Therapist:* What I want to say is that whatever progress Stuart has made has been basically because of you.
>
> *Father:* I don't know.
>
> *Therapist:* I think so, and I think that it's not time to be modest now.
>
> *Father:* I'm not trying to be modest.
>
> *Therapist:* You see, what I'm trying to point out to you, both of you, but basically to you, is that there are a lot of things that are—there are a lot of things that you have done about Stuart's fears [p. 238].

This is particularly important in termination interviews as the practitioner prepares the client for the time interval between this session and the follow-up interview. The helper's effort, of course, is to ensure that the progress that has taken place during intervention will continue (or at least stabilize) during the follow-up interval. Reinforcing the client's sense of mastery, through emphasizing task accomplishment, is a tangible contribution to this process. Quite aside from clinical conviction, there is some suggestive empirical evidence (Liberman, 1978) that the client's positive perception of task accomplishment during treatment tends to promote greater gains at follow-up.

INCREMENTAL CHANGE TASKS

As I pointed out earlier, one of the hazards of natural problem-solving efforts is the tendency to attempt change too rapidly or in a global manner. The struggling individual is sorely tempted to attempt major change "at one blow," the New Year's resolution phenomenon, and the risks of failure of course are great. Tasks in the incremental change category, by contrast, are designed to bring about personal or environmental change in a systematic, step-by-step manner. Such tasks usually follow a hierarchical arrangement, logical or emotional, so as to capitalize on the principle of shaping. The series of tasks utilized with Mrs. Lorenson (see Chapter 3) as she sought to move out of her parental home is an example of this type of task. As Chapter 8, on social skill training, will explicate, many of these educational approaches involve such carefully individualized assignments.

The sequence of tasks employed in sexual therapy (Masters and Johnson, 1970) is an especially clear example of the incremental change task. Although these tasks are usually employed in couple therapy, a mode of intervention this book does not consider, it will be valuable to examine their sequence and rationale. Masters and Johnson (1966) view such sexual dysfunctions as male impotence and female anorgasmia as largely due to a combination of anxiety, faulty sexual communication and technique, and misinformation and ignorance about sexual matters. Along with a number of other instructions, the couple are directed to carry out a series of interrelated homework tasks:

1. Initially the couple's intimate contact is limited to touching and caressing exercises, specifically nonsexual, in order to learn ways of reducing the tension and anxiety that has permeated their

sexual interaction. Additionally, this assignment enables the couple to reexperience the affectionate behaviors which characterized their early relationship before it became specifically sexual.

2. Subsequently, more explicit sexual touching is prescribed, but, as in the previous exercise, the couple are to refrain from orgasmic release. Instead their focus is upon learning ways of increasing sensuality and arousal that are sensitive to their individual needs. Both of these early assignments encourage the development of open verbal communication within a relaxed and nondemanding atmosphere.

3. Further assignments then focus on the partner's learning to stimulate each other to orgasm manually or orally. If the major dysfunction is female anorgasmia, this step in the task sequence capitalizes on the woman's capacity to respond to direct clitoral stimulation, thus promoting the likelihood of satisfying sexual response early in the change process. Where impotence is a major concern, the couple learn alternate methods of sexual gratification that are not dependent upon male erection.

4. Finally, the couple are directed to experiment with coital methods of lovemaking, but even here the assignment is carefully graduated. They are usually directed to employ the female-superior position for intercourse first. This coital position allows for greater female stimulation, if anorgasmia has been problematic, and, in cases of male erectile failure, avoids the coital position (male-superior) where previous failure had most likely occurred.

The gradient of demand and achievement running through this series of tasks is quite apparent. Early tasks ask little of the couple, and with even minimal effort a reasonable degree of success can be attained. Yet at the same time, these initial tasks lay a foundation of tension reduction and enhanced communication that tends to potentiate the accomplishment of the later tasks. Each of the later steps, it will be noted, continues this careful balancing of expectation and potential attainment.

Incremental change tasks often follow what might be called a function–dysfunction or "matching to groups" paradigm. That is to say, where an individual is having difficulty in a particular area, the goal of intervention is to assist this person to become more like those who are considered functional in this same area—to match their performance. This requires that the practitioner have specific knowledge of the characteristics of adequate functioning so that, usually through a series of successive approximations, these characteristics can be replicated in the client. Clear instructions and appropriate models of the desired behaviors at each stage of the learning process are essential.

Identification and sequencing of tasks in sexual therapy have been greatly aided by knowledge of this very sort. Masters and Johnson (1966), in their landmark study of sexual behavior, empirically identified the characteristics of good sexual functioning prior to developing their remedial program for sexual dysfunction. Thus, instead of depending on purely theoretical speculations about sexual behavior, the change process could be clearly related to objective data. Similar considerations will be apparent in the following chapter, where such areas of skill development as assertion training and stress management are discussed. Incremental change assignments, following a carefully gradated sequence of tasks (both inside and out of the therapeutic session), and firm links to empirically derived norms of performance are the *sine qua non* of these approaches.

IMPROVING TASK PERFORMANCE

As a part of his continued effort to establish a firmer empirical base for short-term practice, William Reid (1975) has examined the effects of a carefully devised procedure for increasing client task accomplishment through helper explanation and support. Reid found that with clients seen in mental health and public school settings this procedure significantly increased the probability that tasks would be carried out. Five steps are involved in this Task Implementation Sequence:

1. *Enhancing commitment*. Following assignment of the task the practitioner reviews with the client the potential benefits that could be gained by carrying out the task. Thus the task's potential role in supplying needed information, challenging detrimental beliefs and attitudes, or beginning a process of desired change should be clearly related to the client's anticipated goals.

2. *Planning task implementation*. The clinician must carefully define the specific details of the task including what the client will do and when and where. Any sequence of steps the task might involve is spelled out. The helper should avoid task assignments that are vague or general ("Try to talk to your wife") and, if several steps are involved, should consider whether a more limited task would be more likely to succeed.

3. *Analyzing obstacles*. Client participation is solicited to examine any potential problems that might arise in carrying out the task. For example, negative reactions from significant people in the client's environment should be realistically considered and, if necessary, methods of handling such reactions worked out.

4. *Practice through modeling and behavior rehearsal*. Certain tasks may need to be practiced within the interview, especially where such social skills as clear communication and assertiveness are called for. Feedback from client rehearsal can identify yet another possible point where the task assignment must be modified, especially if the client's facility in the needed skills proves to be low.

5. *Summarizing*. In the final step of the Task Implementation Sequence the helper restates the assigned task and the plan worked out with the client for its implementation. The clinician's expectation that the task will be performed can be underscored by writing it down on a sheet of paper or in the client's notebook (where observational tasks are being recorded) as a reminder.

A recent article by Hepworth (1979) offers some highly useful discussion of the clinical application of the Task Implementation Sequence. Hepworth considers the step of analyzing (and removing) obstacles to be particularly vital in stimulating effective task performance. He points out that, in eliciting potential barriers, the clinician should be alert to the nonverbal cues that could indicate client hesitancy or apprehension:

> Such cues include looking away from the worker, speaking diffi- dently or unenthusiastically in discussing the task, changing the topic, fidgeting atypically, shifting the posture, and tightening facial and body muscles. If such reactions are detected, the worker is well advised to further explore the presence of undisclosed barriers or to work further on resolving obstacles already identified [p. 319].

At the same time Hepworth notes that the helper should not expect that the client who is ready to attempt a task will not feel some degree of apprehension:

> Such readiness, however, should not be confused with feeling comfortable; it is neither realistic nor desirable for the worker to expect the client to feel comfortable with the task. A certain amount of tension and anxiety is to be expected and may positively motivate the client to risk the new behavior embodied in the task [p. 319].

Finally, as noted earlier, carrying out tasks concerned with distressing behavior and emotions may, in some instances, as- sume a paradoxical quality as the clinician directs clients to ob- serve or grapple with the very aspects of their lives that have been most troublesome. Burns and Beck (1978), for example, describe an intensely anxious woman who was referred for therapy but phoned to report that she was afraid to come in even for an initial interview. Her apprehension was that she would pass out on the train as she traveled to the clinic. The therapist discussed these fears with her during the telephone conversation and instructed her to "look for upsetting visual images and frightening thoughts and make notes about these on the train, including a numerical count of the number of such images as well as the content of the fantasies" (p. 127). They note the immediate effects of this as- signment:

> This paradoxical maneuver of instructing the patient to look for and write down these thoughts and fantasies undercut the patient's

fear and avoidance of such anxiety reactions. She appeared in person at the next therapy session and reported that there had been no cognitive or emotional upset since the telephone call, although she had been diligently looking for one! [p. 127]

Haley (1963, 1976) suggests that paradoxical tasks operate through setting up a situation in which the client can rebel against the authority of the therapist only by *not* experiencing the problematic behaviors and emotions. Thus clients who have been instructed to observe certain behaviors can thwart the helper's assumption of control over their lives by reporting that these behaviors did not occur.

However, I believe that a simpler explanation, and one more consonant with the available empirical evidence, is that the client is responding to the demand characteristics or placebo effects implicit in entering a therapeutic relationship. That is to say, the very act of seeking help usually stimulates powerful beliefs and corresponding emotions, implying that relief from suffering will take place. This change in the client's belief system, toward a more hopeful viewpoint, elicits similar changes in behavior and affect. Shapiro and Morris (1978) offer extensive documentation of the effects of such factors in both physical and psychological therapies. Similarly, Bergin and Lambert's (1978) review of the impact of even minimal therapeutic contact suggests that the arousal of more hopeful attitudes is a potent force in personal change. Thus the therapist's assignment of a task concerned with the client's actual difficulties conveys the belief that the client can master these problems and that they need not be avoided. It is immaterial, in a certain sense, whether the client immediately experiences a reduction in problematic behavior—the therapeutic effect comes from fostering a belief that mastery can be attained.

UTILIZING TASKS AND HOMEWORK IN PRACTICE

Directing clients to carry out tasks and homework, as I have frequently emphasized, is a core characteristic of time-limited intervention. It is through the performance of task assignments that much of the personal and behavioral change needed to achieve the goals of therapy is implemented or triggered. In addition, as the preceding chapter stressed, behavioral enactments carried out within the interview are intimately related to this same process. Enactments may suggest potential tasks or, in other instances, are utilized to prepare a client for the implementation of an assignment between sessions. Several other underlying themes are implicit in the utilization of tasks.

At a fundamental level the use of tasks typifies the interest of the brief therapist in bringing about change in the immediate problem the client is experiencing. Asking a client to carry out a task, however minor or peripheral it may appear, conveys to the client how serious the therapist is about the expected outcome of the helping process. The clinician assumes that the client has a similar concern about goal attainment but has had to turn to a professional helping source because of difficulties in mobilizing personal resources or because of a lack of assistance from the people in his or her immediate environment. Requiring the client to behave differently through performing tasks not only suggests the active, goal-oriented nature of brief treatment but offers a direct test of the client's willingness to engage in change attempts.

At the same time, the fact that tasks take place outside the therapeutic session conveys an important message to the clinician as well as to the client. The concept of instigative therapy, as I have already noted, reduces the importance of the therapeutic session and, in its place, highlights the primacy of change in the natural environment. What really matters are the changes that take place in the client's actual life. From this viewpoint, therapist and therapeutic method are only servants to this essential goal. Such a focus tends to reduce client dependency and in addition promotes an important theme of self management or personal coping.

There are some distinct differences between the employment of tasks and the everyday tactic of advice giving that need to be examined at this point. Tasks are assigned within a context in which the practitioner, as the individual prescribing the task, has an explicit mandate—a contract with the client—to bring about some desired type of change. Advice giving, at least in its everyday manifestations, seldom has so clear-cut a sanction. Thus advice is commonly given with such introductory phrases as "Why don't you try . . . ?" or "Have you thought of . . . ?" Task assignment, as the Minuchin transcript illustrates, is unabashedly direct. The therapist simply says, "For this week, I want you to . . . " and spells out the exact nature of the assignment. At times the therapist may employ what Bandler et al. (1976) have called the "polite command" ("What I would like you to do, if you would, is to . . . "), but even here the directive intent of the clinician is clear.

In contrast to advice, then, it is quite apparent that the practitioner expects the task to be carried out. Furthermore, the clinician lets the client know that each assignment will explicitly followed up and, in succeeding sessions, there will be discussion of the salient aspects of the individual's performance, successful or otherwise. Advice, of course, is of a much more tentative nature and is seldom given with anything like these expectations of performance and follow-up.

Finally, a nagging concern for clinicians is how to manage situations in which the client does not carry out an assigned task or, more commonly, only partially completes it. The sensitive and consistent employment of the guidelines discussed earlier (particularly Reid's Task Implementation Sequence) should reduce this possibility, but there is no doubt that it will occur from time to time. In such instances the first consideration the helper must address is the question of task difficulty—was this an assignment that was simply beyond the existing capabilities of the client? If so, how can it be scaled down to a level where satisfactory performance would be possible? The partially completed task is less problematic as its successful elements can be reviewed (and reinforced) and the uncompleted portions can serve as a basis for further assignment. If necessary, the clinician and client must discuss the relevance of the assignment to the goals of therapy *as the client perceives them,* and determine whether the failure to perform was related to some aspect of this issue. Finally, if the client has been consistently neglecting task performance, it may be necessary to review the entire contract between therapist and client to ascertain whether they have the same objectives in working together. In some cases failure to perform tasks may be the client's only way of indicating that he is uncertain or reluctant about change. It is not disastrous to discover and face this important question at a relatively early phase of the therapeutic process rather than continue an endeavor that has little realistic possibility of benefiting the client.

Chapter 8

Teaching for Living: Enhancing Social Skills

These things are important not because a
High-sounding interpretation can be put upon them
But because they are useful.

—Marianne Moore

Difficulties in living frequently involve relationships and interactions with other people that have become troubled or dissatisfying. Wives and husbands are unable to talk together without quarreling, children are bewildered by the demands of their peers, and for many others, young and old, making requests, developing new friendships, and withstanding social pressures have become burdensome and stressful. It has become increasingly common in recent years to regard such difficulties as manifestations of social skill deficits rather than call upon more elaborate explanations. That is to say, troubled individuals are simply seen as never having had the opportunity to learn the requisite social skills required for effective living or as not having developed skills suitable for managing the life situation presently confronting them. The therapeutic task, then, is one of providing education in the particular skills that are missing from the client's repertoire or that have been only haphazardly developed.

Kazdin (1978, p. 67) suggests five potential areas for social skill training:

1. Developing contacts with friends
2. Participating in social groups and activities
3. Finding and keeping employment
4. Developing heterosexual relationships
5. Interacting adequately with family members

As a means of developing facility in these major areas a series of procedures have been devised, largely based upon the shaping, modeling, and positive reinforcement principles of social learning theory. Most practitioners have some familiarity with assertion training, and in marital and family therapy various communication training approaches have enjoyed a minor vogue. In addition, training methods have been developed concerned with such aspects of living as problem solving, job finding, dating and courtship, direct sexual functioning, and stress management. Training has been carried out with adults, adolescents, conflicted marital couples, school children, former mental patients, divorced persons, dating couples, juvenile delinquents, and so on. Given this richness of application and approach, I will arbitrarily limit my discussion in this chapter to three major areas of skill training—assertion training, stress management methods, and heterosocial skill enhancement—and consider how these may be adapted to short-term intervention with troubled individuals.

Each of these training approaches will be described in some detail and illustrated through practice examples. It will be apparent that in some cases the training constituted the major focus of intervention. *However, in other instances, the training was very

---

*This is consonant with Epstein's (1980) position that providing skills is one of the two main procedures of short-term treatment. Epstein considers providing resources as the other major short-term intervention. I can agree with this position as long as one can view the provision of resources in its broadest sense—that is to say, as including not only tangible and concrete services but the more intangible resources of information and education.

specifically focused and formed only a part of a series of interventions.

Assertion Training

Possibly the earliest distinct use of assertion training in clinical practice was described by Andrew Salter in his book *Conditioned Reflex Therapy* (1949). Salter, one of the pioneers of behavior therapy, distinguished between "inhibitory" and "excitatory" behaviors, the latter term coinciding with what we now call assertion. He suggested a series of guidelines for training clients in assertiveness. These priciples are still highly pertinent to clinical practice, and I will return to them later in this section.

Following Salter's work, other early behavior therapists continued the refinement of assertion training techniques. The writings of Wolpe (1973) and Lazarus (Wolpe and Lazarus, 1966) have been particularly influential. At the beginning of the 1970s there was a significant increase in public awareness and interest in the principles of assertiveness and soon a remarkable number of self-help books appeared on the commercial market.* Around the same time feminist writers and therapists recognized that assertive skills were a neglected aspect of female experience, and many women's groups began to incorporate such training (Linehan and Egan, 1978; Jakubowski-Spector, 1973).

Lange and Jakubowski (1976) provide a comprehensive description of assertion training, integrating both behavioral and cognitive constructs, and their work is the most useful available guide for the clinician. They identify four basic procedures in the training process:

(1) Teaching people the differences between assertion and aggression and between nonassertion and politeness; (2) helping people

---

*These include works by Alberti and Emmons (1974), Fensterheim and Baer (1975), and Smith (1975). Such books can serve as valuable reading assignments for clients in the early stages of training.

identify and accept both their own personal rights and the rights of others; (3) reducing existing cognitive and affective obstacles to acting assertively, e.g., irrational thinking, excessive anxiety, guilt, and anger; and (4) developing assertive skills through active practice methods . . . [p. 2].

Initially, however, assertion training must be identified as a reasonable method of reaching the goals the client wishes to achieve or as a useful adjunct to dealing with a particular life difficulty. It is only occasionally that a client will specifically request assertion training. What is more often the case is that the client's target problems involve noticeable difficulties in dealing with some (or all) of the people in his or her immediate environment. The client may view this as due to the intractability or insensitivity of these significant others, and a part of the therapist's task will be to explain how increased assertion could be pertinent to problem resolution. Other clients may be experiencing considerable frustration or anxiety stemming from persistent failure in important interactions. Assertion training may serve as a viable means to the client's goal of gaining relief from the reactive emotional distress. In either case, it must be noted, the brief therapist is not utilizing assertion training as an end in itself or as a substitute for the client's desired goal. Training is employed as a *procedure* specific to achieving the client's chosen goals.

A case illustration, described in the first chapter of this book, will further illuminate the adaptability of assertion training to clinical practice. The reader will recall Mr. Antonini, who was extremely anxious and depressed as a result of the many months of harassment by his fellow workers. This largely consisted of innuendos about his masculinity and suggestions that he was homosexual. Mr. Antonini thought that the difficulties began following an incident when, he believed, he had been overheard masturbating in the factory washroom.

As I pointed out earlier, one of the major interventions was sexual reeducation, as Mr. Antonini's reactions in part were stemming from sexual guilt and confusion. There was also a need to provide him with some direct means of coping with the daily gibes he was enduring. Assertion training appeared to be a potential answer.

Initial exploration of his method of coping with the ridicule revealed that Mr. Antonini generally tended to ignore the remarks or to try to avoid the men who were most active in tormenting him. It was almost inconceivable to him that he could make any direct reply to their sallies. He had thought of physically attacking them, but although he was a relatively husky man, he was apprehensive about the consequences of such direct action.

The therapist explained the difference between aggression and assertion and utilized this explanation as an entry point into exploration of Mr. Antonini's general level of assertion. This was done through a series of hypothetical critical incidents—"What would you do if you bought a shirt at a department store and found it was slightly defective after you returned home?" "How would you go about telling your foreman that you think he's demanding too much work from you?" and so on. These suggested incidents were varied so as to cover a range of situations containing minor to major degrees of stress, and all, of course, were potentially applicable to Mr. Antonini's life context. As Mr. Antonini described his typical reactions to these stressful situations, it became apparent that assertiveness was problematic for him. Although not as unassertive as some clients, he generally tended to handle even mild difficulties through inaction or indirect means.

As the helper described the procedures and goals of assertion training, Mr. Antonini somewhat hesitantly agreed that developing this ability might be helpful to him. He clearly realized that he needed more effective ways of dealing with the harassment and at this point was ready to grasp at any straw. The practitioner was willing to accept this positive, though weak, level of motivation rather than struggle to attain a stronger one. As Hepworth (1979) points out in relation to task performance, *readiness* to attempt an assignment (or in this case a change procedure) should not be confused with a lack of any uncertainty or ambivalence. Early stages in the helping process are often associated with considerable client reluctance.

From the preceding discussion and further brainstorming on existing social situations, a series of incidents were developed in which Mr. Antonini found assertiveness problematic. Wolpe's (1973) Subjective Units of Distress Scale (SUDS) was employed to arrange these into a hierarchy. Like most clients, Mr. Antonini was easily able to grasp the experiential continuum suggested by the SUDS and rate incidents from 5 to 10 (minor tension) up to 90 to 100 (extreme anxiety). This resulted in the following training hierarchy:

SUDS Level	Social Situation
10	—Correcting poor service in a restaurant
15	—Someone cutting into line ahead of him
25	—Asking his foreman for overtime
35	—Stating a differing opinion to his wife
45	—Firmly disciplining his children
50	—Contradicting his mother's opinion
55	—Purchasing prophylactics at a drugstore from a female clerk
60	—Arguing with older men at work
75	—Stating his own opinion with his father
100	—Direct response to harassing sexual remark

These incidents formed the basis for a series of behavior rehearsals during the fourth to seventh sessions of the eight-interview contract with Mr. Antonini. The earlier interviews had been largely concerned with sexual education for both Mr. Antonini and his wife and involved reading assignments, discussion, and specific tasks (adapted from sexual therapy methods) designed to enhance their immediate sexual functioning. Assertion training became highly appropriate as Mr. Antonini's guilt and confusion in sexual matters began to diminish.

The role-plays began with the least demanding situations in Mr. Antonini's hierarchy and, session by session, progressed up this continuum. As his wife attended the sessions, she was asked to play the part of various participants in the enactments; where only therapist and client are available these roles must be shared. The behavior rehearsals usually followed the standard format (see Chapter 6) of enactment–modeling–practice, and Salter's (1949) guidelines were employed to articulate the principles of effective assertion:

Nonverbal dimensions. The client's initial task is to develop such physical aspects of assertiveness as firm voice tone and volume, reasonable eye contact, appropriate bodily stance, and, in general, a freer use of gesture.

Minimal self-disclosure. At a beginning level trainees are encouraged to use the personal pronoun "I" in stating a request or denial, rather than the impersonal phrasings typically employed by the nonassertive person. More revealing levels of self-disclosure are introduced, as appropriate, as training progresses.

Expression of feeling. Rather than employ blaming or defensive responses the client is taught to express the emotional reaction ("I was upset when you did that") engendered by the situation. At early stages of training the level of intensity expected must be carefully guaged in order to avoid alarming the trainee or, in a few instances, promoting aggressiveness.

Improvisation. Throughout the entire sequence of enactments the client is supported in developing a spontaneous and natural style of assertion. The clinician frequently emphasizes that there are no specific formulas for effective living, only general guidelines, but that through practice the client will gain facility in adapting these to a variety of situations. The fact that behavior rehearsals *must* be improvised helps to promote this valuable facet of assertive response.

Expressing disagreement. Unassertive prople often need concentrated practice in expressing disagreement, even within the protective confines of an enactment. Smith's (1975) "broken record" exercise is highly useful in this area. Thus during structured role-play the trainee is allowed to use only a single sentence of disagreement (for example, "No, you can not borrow my car") no matter what tactics the other individual in the enactment may employ. The single phrase must be repeated again and again without qualification or variation. The exercise, which may initially be enacted around hypothetical situations, can have a startling effect in desensitizing the trainee to expressing disagreement.

Expressing (or receiving) positive feelings. The client may need help in directly expressing the positive feelings that are appropriate to a situation, particularly where these must be combined with the assertive denial of a request. Expressing intimate feelings or accepting compliments (without disqualifying oneself) may also be problematic and require attention.

With some clients assertion generally may be adequate but difficulties with a particular person will be evident. In such instances the training hierarchy must concentrate on a graduated series of demands within this troublesome relationship. For example, a middle-aged man found any degree of assertion with his wife extremely difficult, and their relationship was considerably strained by his apparent passivity. The following hierarchy was developed with him and used as a basis for assertion training:

SUDS Level	Relationship Situation
10	—Speaking to wife about messing up bathroom
15	—Asking wife about any of her relatives
25	—Speaking to wife about work she brings home from her job
30	—Asking wife to go to a movie
50	—Asking for help with household chores
60	—Complaining to wife about household disorganization
70	—Handling discussion when wife becomes angry
80	—Discussing wife's medical problems
100	—Responding to wife's threats to leave marriage

Whether broadly or narrowly focused, task assignments are given as training progresses. These are used to test out the level of skill attained or to deal with a specific situation that has been rehearsed in the interview. It is not at all unusual for situations demanding assertiveness to appear almost spontaneously from session to session. This seems to be a matter of the client's having developed both greater awareness and increased confidence so that previously avoided situations are now noticed. However, the client should be cautioned agained undertaking an encounter that is too far above the hierarchy level practiced in the session although, generally speaking, overreaching themselves is not a common characteristic of the unassertive. The more likely difficulty is one of motivating task performance, but careful attention to a gradient of assignment usually circumvents this problem.

Observational tasks can be employed at early phases of training to augment its effects. Clients are instructed to observe and record in a notebook the assertive, nonassertive, and aggressive actions they encounter among their friends and associates. An assignment of this kind can help the fearful or pessimistic client to realize that assertiveness not only is possible but does not have dire consequences. Thoughtful observation and analysis of the style of assertive friends and acquaintances can also offer clients an important model, drawn from their own immediate milieu, for further study and emulation.

Assertion training with Mr. Antonini concluded at the eighth session of the agreed-upon intervention. By that time he not only had worked through the less problematic situations on his hierarchy but had rehearsed several appropriately assertive responses to different versions of the harassment. He and his wife were seen in a follow-up interview five months later and reported that his work situation was quite satisfactory. Not only was he no longer being harassed but, as it turned out, he had never had to make any direct response to his co-workers' ridicule, despite being prepared to do so. Apparently his generally enhanced assertiveness, evident through his general manner and physical bearing, had been sufficient to dispell the difficulties.

Stress Management Methods

Like assertion training, the notion of stress management is currently receiving considerable public exposure, particularly in the self-help literature. However, despite their great usefulness self-help manuals are often not a sufficient guide for many people, and a surprising number of individuals are not exposed to such material. The average client's knowledge of stress management or assertion training methods is likely to be scanty and limited to a vague notion that there are ways of dealing with these difficulties.

As Benson (1974) points out, rapid technological change, along with the growing complexity of Western living, has made emotional stress an almost accepted aspect of life. Although many people understand the harmful consequences of stress, few know how to alleviate it. The family physician's common injunction "You've got to learn how to relax" is more a source of frustration to the troubled individual than a helpful directive. How can one possibly put this useful piece of advice into operation?

Training in stress management (Vattano, 1974) usually begins with a survey of the various life situations in which the client finds that uncomfortable tension is developing. A number of clients are able to identify where undue stress is affecting their lives, but some are less aware of this factor and cling to other explanations. The therapist should be alert to the possibility that tension is affecting the client's behavior in critical situations.

Mrs. Loniero, age thirty-seven, returned for individual counseling two years after she and her husband had been seen in marital therapy. In the previous contact only slight improvement had occurred in their long-standing difficulties. Mrs. Loniero described a deteriorating situation in which her husband had resumed heavy drinking and she was now seriously considering divorce. At the same time she spoke of her own anxiety and fear about making this decision and how she was finding herself becoming isolated from friends and experiencing many perturbing physical reactions. Her family physician had found no organic difficulties and had made the usual prescription of Valium. It appeared highly likely that stress management training would be a necessary supplement to meeting her request for help in evaluating her decision to seek a divorce.

Similar needs will be evident where the individual, despite adequate facility in certain areas, repetitively experiences difficulty or failure in managing important social interactions. Finally, behavioral signals such as tightened facial muscles, rigid body posture, fidgety movements, sighs, and pronounced expulsion of breath may be immediately apparent within the interview and lead the practitioner to query the presence of dysfunctional levels of stress.

As in other areas of skill training the helper attempts to develop a common conceptualization with the client during this initial phase. That is to say, client and therapist need to reach a mutual understanding that stress reactions are playing a significant role in the client's difficulties and that training in tension reduction methods seems to be a reasonable approach to dealing with this problem. Explanation from the therapist concerning the effect of stress on human functioning adds to this development of understanding, and along with these more general explanations the educationally oriented therapist usually provides the client with a clear but succinct description of the training process. In contrast to less specific methods of treatment, the social skill training approaches have the enormous advantage of readily lending themselves to concise, nonmystical explanation.

Training in stress management emphasizes three major phases: (1) developing awareness of stress signals, (2) gaining facility in relaxation procedures, and (3) practicing coping with actual stress situations.

Thus as a part of the initial survey of stressful situations the clinician assists the client in identifying how he or she typically displays stress. This may be through specific physical manifestations, through repetitive worrisome thoughts and fantasies, or through vague but powerful anxiety experiences. Whatever their form, these reactions are pinpointed and reinterpreted by the clinician, not as events to be dreaded, but as the necessary signals from body and mind that stress management is required.

Several approaches to tension reduction have been described in the literature and, singly or in combination, can be taught to the client during the second stage of stress management training. Although relaxation training has been presented in some instances as an elaborate procedure, Marks (1978) reviews several empirical studies which suggest that relatively abbreviated methods offer the client as much as the more extended versions.

1. Drawing upon Jacobson's (1929) seminal work on the physiology of muscular tension, a series of exercises has been developed for inducing relaxation in each of the many muscle groups throughout the body. The therapist verbally guides the client through this procedure within the session and then assigns similar exercises as daily homework. It can be helpful to provide the client with an audiotape of the instructions to use in the home practice sessions. Goldfried and Davison (1976) discuss this approach in detail and offer several versions of the relaxation induction process. The clinician should practice this process prior to utilizing it with clients and tape-record these initial attempts. This will offer useful feedback for developing convincing voice tone and verbal fluency and additionally provide the helper with a beneficial appreciation of the immediate effects of the process.

2. Whether or not one places specific emphasis on muscular relaxation, a number of cognitive and physical cues can be built into the induction process. These include key words ("relax," "calm," "gentle"), visual images of pleasant scenes (a sunny day or an idyllic beach), and a concentrated awareness of breathing. I have found it useful initially to employ a relaxation induction process during the session that combines attention to the various muscle groups along with these other cues. From discussion of this experience and further home practice, clients identify the methods that are most useful to them in reducing tension.

3. Finally, a simple meditative method can be taught to the client and, as in the other procedures, further facility gained through daily practice. Benson (1974) has popularized an effective version of this approach:

> In a quiet environment, sit in a comfortable position.
> Close your eyes.
> Deeply relax all your muscles, beginning at your feet and pro-

gressing up to your face—feet, calves, thighs, lower torso, chest, shoulders, neck, head. Allow them to remain deeply relaxed.

Breathe through your nose. Become aware of your breathing. As you breathe out, say the word "one" silently to yourself. Thus: breath in . . . breathe out, with "one." In . . . out, with "one.". . .

Continue this practice for 20 minutes. You may open your eyes to check the time, but do not use an alarm. When you finish, sit quietly for several minutes, at first with your eyes closed and later with your eyes open [p. 74].

Throughout this portion of the training the necessity of systematic practice in tension reduction is consistently emphasized with the client. Daily practice is needed in order to develop a beginning sense of mastery of the method and, importantly, to identify the aspects of the tension reduction process which most reliably induce relaxation for the individual client. Some individuals find cue words most beneficial, others respond best to meditative or visual signals, and so on. The clinician points out that this is an individual matter that can only be determined through consistent practice.

As clients gain facility in inducing relaxation in the practice situation, they are encouraged to begin testing out this facility in real-life encounters. An emphasis is placed on *unobtrusive* means of reducing stress, and the client's ability to employ cue words or breathing devices becomes especially relevant. However, the clinician should point out that complete control of stress is neither necessary nor desirable. As I noted earlier, the client's own stress reactions of worry or various physical manifestations must be used as signals for the employment of stress management. In this sense, a certain level of stress is needed in order to trigger the appropriate coping mechanisms. Indeed, the theme of *coping more successfully* should be highlighted at various stages of the intervention, as this constitutes the most realistic goal of training.

Stress management training, like the other skill enhancement approaches, can constitute the major intervention with certain clients while with others it may be employed to augment other change strategies. In the extended illustrations given in Chapter

3, for example, an adaptation of stress management training was the core intervention in helping Mr. Jurecko to control his anger outbursts. However, with Mr. Faber and Mr. Toman, it will be recalled, relaxation exercises were highly useful but peripheral to other interventions. A further practice illustration will demonstrate this potentiating effect:

> Mr. and Mrs. Thompson, a lower-middle-class couple in their early thirties, were seen for short-term sexual counseling. The major dysfunction was Mrs. Thompson's inability to achieve orgasm. They were initially quite responsive to the structured exercises in the sexual therapy regime. However, it soon became evident that Mrs. Thompson was experiencing considerable stress in her daily work as a beautician and that the relaxation components of the sexual counseling exercises were not sufficient to reduce this factor. Portions of two sessions were then devoted to individual training for her in stress management. Following some practice, this additional intervention was successful in diminishing the extraneous pressures that had been interfering with sexual function.

It should be noted that this additional change strategy had effects in an area other than the problem area directly contracted with Mr. and Mrs. Thompson. That is to say, Mrs. Thompson became much more comfortable and functional in her work, as well as sexually. Thus, although the focused nature of short-term treatment calls for a deliberate restriction in intervention, there is no reason that, from time to time, change strategies introduced to achieve a desired effect will not convey benefits elsewhere. The brief therapist, however, does not indulge in such excursions for their own sake but only if, as with this couple, they are manifestly required to attain the chosen goal.

Heterosocial Skill Enhancement

In an extensive review of the research and clinical work in this area, Galassi and Galassi (1978) define heterosocial skills as "the skills relevant to initiating, maintaining and terminating a social and/or sexual relationship with a member of the opposite sex'' (p. 131). They point out that competence in intimate communication and behavior is considered an essential aspect of adolescent and young adult development and, conversely, that heterosocial problems have been identified as important precursors of later social and emotional difficulty. Although much of the research has been conducted with college student populations and therefore generalization must be cautious, heterosocial problems are undoubtedly a significant area of concern for many individuals.

The case illustration with Mr. Faber (see Chapter 3) involved an extensive use of this approach, while elements of the training were incorporated into the work with Mr. Toman, particularly after he and his wife physically separated. These two individuals are typical of the client populations who can benefit from such training—that is, those, like Mr. Faber, who have lacked adequate family models for learning heterosocial skills or who, like Mr. Toman, are reentering the social arena after a considerable absence. In the latter regard not only the newly divorced but individuals who have been institutionalized, suffered incapacitating illness, or grown up in a different culture can be potential candidates for heterosocial training. Unfortunately most of the research and clinical exploration has been with the problems experienced by shy and inadequate males, to the almost total neglect of the troubled woman. A difficulty in developing effective intervention for women may lie in the prevalent social norms that still require females to play a more passive role in initiating intimate relationships.*

Galassi and Galassi (1978) identify four major theoretical con-

---

*Curiously, the exact reverse of this dilemma exists in sexual therapy, where *individual* sexual counseling with women has been highly successful in dealing with their major dysfunction of anorgasmia (for example, Barbach, 1980). On the other hand, individual work with men, around the common dysfunction of secondary impotence, has been generally discouraging and consequently neglected (LoPiccolo and LoPiccolo, 1978). It appears that in this instance the societal expectation of an assertive role for men operates to their detriment.

structs underlying the approach and suggest that clinical intervention should selectively combine elements from each of these
areas:

Conditioned anxiety. In certain instances the individual, as a
result of unpleasant or difficult intimate experiences, has become
conditioned to avoiding them. The cues associated with close
relationships arouse anxiety, and in such cases treatment may
involve the use of systematic desensitization. At the least, clients
often need some training in stress management in order to cope
with current tensions.

Skill deficits. From this perspective, the lack of specific social
skills impairs the person's performance and consequently leads to
reactive anxiety and avoidance of intimate situations. Clinically
the goal of treatment is to identify the deficient skills and,
through shaping, modeling, and *in vivo* practice, remediate these
gaps.

Cognitive disortions. Galassi and Galassi (1978) note that a
number of individuals have the capability of competent response
but "because of negative self-evaluation (Bandura, 1969), excessively high performance standards, unrealistic expectations,
faulty perceptions, or misinterpretation of feedback, they either
fail to perform or underestimate their performance" (p. 153).
Specific cognitive change procedures will not be considered in
this section but are discussed in greater depth in Chapter 9.

Physical attractiveness. Finally, heterosocial difficulties may
be influenced by the individual's degree of physical attractiveness
or, to reiterate the importance of cognitive mediation, the person's *self-evaluation* of these qualities. Clinical programs should
include some direct (and realistic) focus on this variable.

The work with Mr. Faber, described in Chapter 3, combined
elements from all of these areas. Initially he was given social skill
training in intimate communication and, of course, in a number
of the practical aspects of seeking out increased contact with
women and asking for dates. Further training emphasized various
facets of dating behavior and was integrated with the sexual information provided to ease his anxiety in that critical dimension.

As Galassi and Galassi (1978) point out, the most difficult aspects of dating for both men and women are "finding dates, initiating contact with prospective dates, initiating sexual activity, avoiding or curtailing sex, and ending a date" (p 136). A combination of assertive and communicative skills, as well as a good deal of factual and normative information, must be blended into the training. Aspects of his physical appearance were directly discussed with Mr. Faber, and as the relationship developed, he was firmly guided in taking better care of his personal hygiene and dress. Finally, when the augmentation of his skill deficits and physical appearance proved insufficient to maintain his new relationships, a further series of sessions was utilized to work on both cognitive factors and better stress management.

Applications in Practice

Social skill training has the reputation among some practitioners of being mundane and unexciting and, further, applicable only to highly dysfunctional individuals such as the formerly institutionalized mental patient. In certain senses this reputation is deserved: in comparison with the excitement and mystery evoked by intrapsychic exploration or the feeling of power experienced in devising and applying paradoxical interventions, skill training follows a very routine and orderly course. There is no denying the profound simplicity of its procedures and goals. Helping someone to deal with a prying neighbor or an overbearing employer or to manage the everyday strains of living is very ordinary stuff. Yet this very direct relevance of social skill training to frequent problems in living constitutes its power and makes selected forms of training an often essential component in brief treatment.

The imaginative therapist will find any number of uses for skill training, especially when combined with other interventive methods. In many instances, for example, the client will not need complete assertion training but enough help to be distinctly assertive in an identifiably difficult situation.

Mrs. Anton, a twenty-three-year-old college student, was striving to emancipate herself from a highly dependent yet conflictful relationship with her widowed mother. Many issues concerning her father's death, her mother's recurrent illnesses, and her own values and attitudes as a daughter were related to this struggle.

Careful exploration and reflective discussion of her reactions and responses within the immediate relationship with her mother formed the major intervention and proved helpful. However, as this aspect of treatment progressed, Mrs. Anton felt helpless in contending with her mother's frequent late-night telephone calls and the lengthy, exhausting conversations that ensued. Assertion training was initiated, entirely focused on how to firmly terminate such calls, and behaviorally rehearsed over portions of a session or two. This was sufficient to manage this particularly frustrating aspect of the relationship while work on other areas continued.

In another instance stress management training was utilized as part of a four-session intervention with a woman who was involved in a series of medical tests to determine the extent of a potentially serious physical condition. The training enabled her to cope with her immediate anxiety and additionally freed her to put energy into such tasks as obtaining full information from her physician and evaluating the treatment options available. In a women's health center, yet another creative practitioner used an extremely brief form of the stress management approach to ease the tensions of mentally retarded women about to undergo a gynecological examination. This intervention was all the more remarkable for being implemented in the only time available— during the fifteen or twenty minutes of a preexamination screening interview.

Finally, although I am not directly considering group approaches in this work, it should at least be briefly noted that skill training is easily adaptable to this modality (Rose, 1977). Indeed, assertion training is probably more frequently conducted in groups than as a one-to-one intervention. Many other variations are possible.

As part of a community mental health center's outreach service to an inner-city area, teachers in a junior high school were asked to identify preadolescent boys who were difficult to manage in the classroom or playground. Ten boys, twelve to thirteen years in age, were recruited and assigned to two short-term skill training groups, each lasting seven sessions. Training concentrated on the development of assertive and communicative skills (Gittellman, 1965) in a variety of social situations, using modeling and role-play procedures. The boys were highly participant in this very specific, carefully structured approach, and teacher evaluations (using a standardized rating form) indicated significantly better school adjustment at the conclusion of training.

Such children have often been treated in more loosely structured groups in which it is believed that verbal discussion, recreational activities, and, in general, identification with the group leaders will promote beneficial changes in social adjustment. The skill training approach is an attempt to *directly* focus on imparting the relevant behaviors rather than hope they will arise through less direct means.

Chapter 9

Cognitive Restructuring Methods

And thus the native hue of resolution
Is sicklied o' er with the pale cast of thought.
— William Shakespeare, *Hamlet*

In earlier discussion I pointed out that human experience can be conceptualized along three major dimensions—behavior, emotion, and cognition. The mainstream practice theories have each tended to accentuate one of these facets to the neglect of the others. The behavioral therapists, most obviously, have concentrated upon specific and tangible aspects of motoric activity and, from this base, developed a series of interventive strategies intended to influence this aspect of human functioning. The humanistic and existential approaches have stressed the primacy of emotion and, particularly in their emphasis on the development of an intimate helping relationship, highlighted the place of feelings in the change process. Psychodynamically influenced therapists have been especially interested in the thought patterns, real or fantasied, that affect human relationships and have directed much of their effort toward promoting greater awareness of these forces.

This would obviously be the place to recount the story of the blind men attempting to describe the elephant, but I will spare the reader yet another version of that hoary fable. Suffice it to say, there is ample evidence (Bandura, 1977b) that each of these facets of the human experience, alone or in interaction, is important. This chapter, however, will deliberately isolate a single element, attempting to review recent developments in the cognitive approaches to psychotherapy and the clinical applications of these intriguing theoretical and technical advances.

The notion that cognitions—our thoughts, beliefs, attitudes, and values—can affect our emotions and actions is scarcely new. Both common knowledge and a variety of psychological theories have stressed this relationship. However, although widely espoused, these viewpoints have been rather general, and at a therapeutic level it has been difficult to identify *what* cognitions need to be changed and *how* such change can be most effectively and efficiently accomplished. The development of a number of cognitively oriented therapies over the past decade has materially altered this picture.

In recent years the behavior therapists have been particularly active in devising techniques specifically aimed at cognitive change, and interestingly, these developments hold some promise of a rapprochement between the behavioral and nonbehavioral approaches. A number of clinicians from other orientations have also significantly contributed to this trend. In contrast to previous approaches, the emerging cognitive therapies have been marked by several distinctive features (Mahoney and Arkoff, 1978):

1. An emphasis on the specific identification of intruding or detrimental cognitive processes as *current* factors in the person's functioning
2. The development of discrete techniques for inducing change in these factors
3. A general emphasis on cognitive change as a *procedure,* rather than an end in itself

This last feature is especially consonant with the emphasis of short-term therapy on the primacy of change efforts aimed at the client's selected problem in living. That is to say, cognitive change should not be sought for its own sake, but cognitive techniques can be utilized, alone or in combination with other strategies, toward the contracted goals of the intervention. The issue for the practitioner, therefore, is whether achieving change in a target problem such as a conflicted relationship or reactive emotional distress can be most efficiently and effectively attained through a cognitively oriented intervention or through some other strategy.

The practitioner interested in cognitive change procedures will soon become aware that, as in almost any area of psychotherapeutic endeavor, there are numerous cognitive approaches available. In the empirical and pluralistic spirit emphasized in this book, these differences will be regarded as complementary rather than competitive. The available research evidence will be considered, and the usefulness of these many strategies to the immediate purposes of brief intervention will be evaluated.

Four major theoretical constructs utilized in the cognitive therapies will be reviewed, and the supporting references for each of these will suggest further readings for the interested practitioner. Initially I will examine the social learning theory concept of self-efficacy, regarding this construct as the central factor in both cognitive and behavioral change. Succeeding sections will review the cognitive theory and practice related to irrational beliefs, faulty thinking processes, and inhibiting or facilitating self-dialogues. In the concluding sections of the chapter some further cognitive change techniques will be described and illustrated.

Efficacy Assumptions

In outlining the immediate goals of the initial interview (see Chapter 4), I suggested that arousing hope was the primary objective of the early engagement process. At that point I referred to Bandura's (1977b) discussion of efficacy expectations and suggested that the individual's belief in his own competence to act was an essential ingredient of hope. Bandura has continued, both theoretically and empirically, to examine this central construct and indeed has produced persuasive evidence that changes in self-efficacy are closely related to all forms of personal and behavioral change. From this viewpoint the effectiveness of *any* therapeutic procedure is governed by its ability to heighten the troubled individual's sense of competence.

To reiterate, Bandura (1977a) differentiates between two types of expectancy belief. He defines an *outcome expectancy* as "a person's estimate that a given behavior will lead to certain outcomes" (p. 193). For example, I may consider it most likely that I will receive a raise in salary if I directly request this of my employer. On the other hand, an *efficacy assumption* is "the conviction that one can successfully execute the behavior required to produce the outcomes" (p. 193). In relation to the previous example, I may have only a low level of belief in my actual ability to make such a direct request. Certain consequences can follow from the individual's perceived self-efficacy:

> The strength of people's convictions in their own effectiveness is likely to affect whether they will even try to cope with given situations . . . . People fear and tend to avoid threatening situations they believe exceed their coping skills, whereas they get involved in activities and behave assuredly when they judge themselves capable of handling situations that would otherwise be intimidating [Bandura, 1977a, pp. 193–194].

As a central mediator between information and action, self-efficacy is also seen as influencing coping efforts once they are underway. Higher levels of perceived self-efficacy will tend to promote greater persistence and strength in the individual's coping behavior. Lower levels are more likely to result in inhibition or failure and, consequently, perpetuation of the perceived incompetence. Bandura notes, however, that "expectation alone will not produce desired performance if the component capabilities are lacking" (p. 194), and as the preceding chapter stressed, the troubled individual may need careful training in any of a series of deficient social skills in order to raise his or her perception of self-efficacy and make action even possible.

The social learning analysis identifies four major sources of information about efficacy, each of which corresponds with certain clinical procedures. The most powerful of these sources are *performance accomplishments,* that is to say, actions of the individual that demonstrate the ability to cope. Next in potency are what Bandura calls *vicarious experiences,* in which the person sees others coping successfully with similar problems. It is also possible to gain a heightened level of self-efficacy through the *verbal persuasion* provided by significant others (including, of course, the therapist), although this source of information is generally weaker in its effects because of the lack of genuine participation by the individual. Finally, certain forms of *emotional arousal* can add to self-efficacy perceptions, particularly if the person finds that the aroused emotion in a feared situation is less debilitating than had been anticipated.

Bandura and his associates (1977a, 1980) have conducted a series of studies within the psychotherapeutic setting to determine the generality of self-efficacy theory and to identify the comparative strength of these various approaches to altering the individual's perceptions. Their data substantiate that perceived self-efficacy is closely related to therapeutic gain and, furthermore, changes in concert with a variety of behavioral and other measures. In examining changes in clients with severely disabling phobias, for example, they found that enactive therapeutic methods, particularly those emphasizing real-life tasks, were most beneficial in increasing self-efficacy. These studies of therapeutic process strongly suggest that the major aim of any intervention must be to heighten perceived self-efficacy and that methods that stimulate the individual's actual performance accomplish this objective most effectively.

Although these conclusions are generally supportive of such typical behavioral approaches as modeling and desensitization, the implications of the data are much broader. For example, the emphasis of short-term therapy on behavior enactment and task assignment is supported by these findings; these methods are shown not simply as convenient short-cuts toward change, but as critically related to the need to induce change in the client's sense of competence. Both of these methods are enactive and, when skillfully shaped to the client's immediate needs, can provide the necessary foundation for this key aspect of cognitive change. As later sections of this chapter will describe, tasks are frequently employed in all of the major cognitive therapies.

This is not to say that therapeutic procedures involving verbal persuasion or emotional arousal should not be employed. At many points throughout this work I have suggested ways in which the therapist can utilize language or, in other instances, the nuances of the immediate relationship as a part of the helping art. However, it is apparent that the effect of these techniques on a central construct such as self-efficacy is relatively weak and methods that solely rely on such strategies would be questionable, particularly where the troubled individual is struggling with a problem of some magnitude. Thus such techniques as redefinition, relabeling, suggestion, supplying information, reshaping attribution, and so on are best regarded as supplementary to such active strategies as modeling, behavior rehearsal, and task performance. The various forms of emotional arousal, such as ventilation, catharsis, confrontation, and the like, should be seen in a similar light. They form a useful part of the therapeutic repertoire but are most effective when preparatory to, or combined with, the active strategies that can directly foster heightened competence or self-efficacy.

Irrational Beliefs

Perhaps the earliest and best known of the cognitive approaches is Albert Ellis's (1962, 1971) rational-emotive therapy (RET). Ellis has contended that certain strongly held beliefs intervene within the troubled person and either arouse such negative emotions as anxiety or depression or severely impair the individual's judgment and ability to act. In either case, effective management of even normal problems in living is profoundly affected.

Ellis calls these beliefs "irrational ideas" and has identified a set of twelve that he regards as most detrimental as well as most commonly held by troubled people. These include, for example, the belief that "it is a dire necessity for an adult human being to be loved or approved by virtually every significant other person in his community" (1962, p. 61), that "one should be thoroughly competent, adequate, and achieving in all possible respects, if one is to consider oneself worthwhile" (1962, p. 63), and "the idea that it is awful and catastrophic when things are not the way one would very much like them to be" (1962, p. 69). These three appear to be the most fundamental of the irrational ideas. The remainder, as Lange and Jakubowski (1976) suggest, can probably be considered " 'second order' cognitive reactions after one of the three basic beliefs is operating" (p. 127).

The RET approach to cognitive modification includes (1) identifying the irrational assumptions most affecting the client, (2) convincing the client of the potency of these beliefs in his or her life, (3) verbally challenging the logic of the client's irrational belief system, and (4) further exercises and assignments, both in the interview and outside, to develop a more rational belief system. DiLoreto (1971) offers empirical data from a carefully designed controlled study on the efficacy of the RET approach.

Two aspects of RET are particularly worth noting. First, the theoretical principles of the approach are immediately and openly taught to the client, usually in the initial phases of intervention. It is considered essential that the individual have a clear grasp of the RET cosmology in order to be able to examine and change his or her life in accord with these principles. However, perhaps the unique feature of the RET approach to cognitive change is the frequent use of a technique of direct disputation in relation to the client's irrational beliefs. The therapist persistently challenges these assumptions, utilizing a combination of probing questions and pointed confrontations, along with continued teaching of

RET theory and philosophy. Walen et al. (1980) offer many examples of this strategy. Here is one:

> *Client:* But it's awful if I don't get this promotion!
> *Therapist:* Well, just how is that so awful?
> *Client:* Because ... then I'll be stuck in the same job and I won't get the extra money nor the prestige that goes with it.
> *Therapist:* Look, Jack, that's evidence for why it's unfortunate or bad that you don't get the promotion. Because it's bad, it doesn't follow that it's terrible. Now, try again. Can you show me how it's *terrible?*
> *Client:* But I've worked hard for this for a long time. I deserve it!
> *Therapist:* Jack, that may be true that you've worked hard. But that's only further evidence that it's unfortunate that you didn't get it. How is that *terrible?*
> *Client:* You mean all those reasons for it being bad don't make it terrible?
> *Therapist:* That's right, Jack! Terrible means you can't live with this or possibly be happy. It means 101 percent bad. Now, how is failing to get the promotion *that bad?* [p. 100]

Walen et al. (1980) discuss the disputation method in some detail and provide the practitioner with many useful guidelines for its application. Their discussion is also noteworthy for its examination of many of the nuances of the directive approach in therapy, an often neglected dimension of therapeutic activity.

Irrational ideas can also be challenged and altered through homework assignments. Some examples of these were briefly reviewed in Chapter 7 when risk-taking and shame-attacking assignments were discussed. Yet another instance involved a young man struggling with moderate depression as he attempted to work out more adequate personal relationships. Discussion revealed that he was convinced that almost everyone else, unlike him, was happy and contented. This belief had the effect of generating a good deal of inhibiting rumination and self-pity. He was instructed to ask several of his friends and acquaintances whether they were happy and to listen carefully to their replies. The following week he reported his amazement at the amount of discontent this simple question had revealed, placing his own troubles in a much more realistic perspective.

Faulty Thinking Processes

The individual is constantly engaged in processing the information received from various external and internal sources, and in the course of such operations many errors may arise. Mistakes in judgment then ensue and, from these, maladaptive behaviors may result. Such writers as Beck (1976), Mahoney (1974), and Raimy (1975) have contributed to the theoretical base and the clinical applications of this approach to cognitive restructuring. Its resemblance, of course, to many of the tenets of ego psychology will also be apparent.

Rathjen et al. (1978) suggest that from a clinical perspective the essential question in relation to cognitive processing is "What underlying rules lead to competent and incompetent performance?" (p. 42). Each of us, at any given moment, receives information from many sources—the opinions and actions of others, cues from the immediate physical environment, our own emotional and physiological reactions, and stray recollections of past experiences, to name only a few. These must be interpreted, encoded, evaluated, and, when needed, recalled in order to make a decision or mobilize a particular action. Arriving at a decision or carrying out an action, in turn, provides further information which must be managed in the same way.

Governing this process are a series of underlying rules, often quite idiosyncratic, that are utilized to organize and simplify what would otherwise be an overwhelming mass of data. The cognitive therapists have identified a series of common errors or distortions in cognitive processing that may seriously mar its operation, and these are discussed at length by Beck (1976), Burns and Beck

(1978), and Mahoney (1974). A few of the more prominent distortions will be reviewed here.*

Selective inattention. Although the individual must necessarily simplify many aspects of experience, this aspect of the cognitive process can become skewed and involve a neglect of important cues. For example, nonverbal or contextual qualifications can be disregarded in evaluative feedback from significant others, or in other instances the presence of positive statements will be ignored.

Incorrect labeling. On the other hand, information from the environment may be accurately received by mistakenly categorized or labeled by the person. Nonverbal cues are particularly subject to such misclassification as they are by their very nature ambiguous ("Did her silence mean consent?"). Individuals may also mislabel their own internal experiences and, as Walen et al. (1980) point out, misidentify anxiety as guilt or vice versa.

Arbitrary inference. This, of course, is the classic *non sequitur* in which the conclusions do not follow from the premises. More specifically, individuals may reach a conclusion where the available evidence is very scanty or where the evidence is actually contrary to the conclusions drawn.

Magnification. Accurate information processing is heavily dependent on the interpretation the person places on an event. A common error is to exaggerate the personal significance of a current or past experience, thus increasing its potential for dysfunctional emotional arousal.

Overgeneralization. A pernicious tendency in the distressed person is to take a single incident of difficulty or failure as proof of complete personal inadequacy. As in some instances of arbi-

---

*Although I will emphasize how faulty thinking processes affect troubled individuals, it will be obvious that any of these distortions can be present in the processing operations of quite functional people. The misperceptions and erroneous judgments they promote are simply less disastrous for those of us not in an already stressful situation.

trary inference, the critical incident may have some relevance to the issue of adequacy, but its utilization as complete proof is far too general. This kind of fallacious reasoning is particularly likely if the individual has already magnified the importance of the event.

Dichotomous reasoning. In this type of faulty processing, individuals tend arbitrarily to interpret their experience in an either/or fashion. Thus one is either good or bad, lovable or unlovable, and events are joyous or catastrophic, with, no gradations between.

Misplaced attribution. Troubled individuals may tend to ascribe responsibility to external sources in the case of success and to themselves in the case of failure, in both instances significantly impairing their sense of self-efficacy.

The cognitive therapists have developed a variety of approaches to altering these faulty thinking processes. As in any therapeutic approach, the development of a common conceptualization between helper and client concerning the nature and source of the difficulties is essential. It is little use attempting to correct a client's distorted thinking processes if, say, the client is convinced that her problems are due to her husband's insensitivity or the deprivations of her early life.

Burns and Beck (1978) present several case illustrations of their cognitive approach to such mood disorders as depression and anxiety, and in each of these the therapist places considerable emphasis on explaining to the client in simple, straightforward terms how behavior and emotion are affected by thought. These are clinical examples of the structuring techniques described in Chapter 5 and are also closely related to the information-giving function of the therapist, to be discussed later in this chapter. In any case, clients need to grasp the notion that how they are thinking, the manner in which they interpret the information available to them, can profoundly affect both emotional response and behavior. Like any new level of awareness, gaining such knowledge can induce a degree of change, but the helper is well advised not to rely on this alone. The cognitive therapists reinforce and augment such intellectual changes through a series of observational and performance tasks.

Thus logs and diaries are used as a medium for gathering data on the client's immediate experience and the manner in which he or she is processing this information. The Daily Record of Dysfunctional Thoughts (described in Chapter 7) is a prime example of this approach, as the client is encouraged to track the occurrence of disturbing cognitions and in addition to experiment with substituting positive thoughts. At other points the clinician may ask the client to observe and record the presence of errors and distortions in information processing as these actually occur. Finally, material from the client's diary or log can be reviewed within the therapeutic session and faulty thinking patterns directly challenged by the practitioner in a manner analogous to the disputing techniques of the RET advocates.

Lazarus and Fay (1975) offer many examples of cognitively oriented performance tasks in their book *I Can If I Want To*. Although it was written as a popular self-help book, it contains many specific illustrations of tasks that can be utilized by the clinician to influence faulty thinking processes or crippling beliefs. For example, with the individual fearful of making mistakes a series of behavioral assignments might be prescribed including deliberately drawing attention to one's mistakes instead of covering them up, telling friends about certain major mistakes, and keeping a daily log of errors or efforts to conceal mistakes. Similarly, Burns and Beck (1978) not only give an anxious young man the assignment of attending a social gathering but additionally work out a series of related questions on which he is to gather data while at this event in order to test out whether there is any validity to his anticipatory apprehensions about how others will respond to him.

Self-Dialogues: Negative and Positive

Quite aside from these broader concepts of expectation, belief, and cognitive process, there is no doubt that we all have thoughts of many kinds. Distinctly or vaguely, in fragmentary form or in complete phrases and sentences, words flash through our minds as we carry out our daily activities. Meichenbaum (1974, 1975) argues that behavior is mediated by internal cues, often in the form of subvocal dialogues. He distinguishes two varieties of this kind of cognitive mediation, either of which may result in dysfunctional response and consequently difficulties in living:

1. Individuals may be habitually producing a series of *negative* cues in their self-talk which inhibit, block, or disrupt the needed response. For example, in a situation calling for an assertive action the internal dialogue ("I can't do it," "I'll blow it again," "I'm such a fool") may effectively inhibit the desired behavior or at least arouse emotion with much the same effect.

2. On the other hand, individuals may not be providing themselves with the *positive* cognitive cues ("Try that first and see if it works," "Take it easy, you're doing all right") needed to guide, monitor, and encourage a complex behavior. For example, some hyperactive children do not offer themselves the discriminative and self-reinforcing cues necessary for even simple tasks. One of the therapeutic applications of this cognitive construct offers an alternative to the psychopharmocological approaches often utilized in work with such children.

Negative self-dialogues or the lack of positive self-guidance can be particularly disruptive in important interpersonal relationships. With conflicted marital couples, for example, either of these patterns may be operating. A couple can be functioning in terms of negative stereotypes or cues ("He won't listen," "She doesn't care," "I'll just get hurt again") that disrupt such positive actions as affectional gestures and clear requests. On the other hand, through inadequate learning experiences or long-continued conflict, they may also lack the positive discriminative cues ("She'll enjoy this" or "Try to say it more clearly") necessary for maintaining a consistent relationship.

Certain of the principles of systematic densensitization, a therapeutic procedure well established as an effective intervention with severe anxiety (Kazdin and Wilson, 1978(, have been adapted to the treatment of negative self-dialogues. Meichen-baum calls this approach *self-instructional training* (SIT) because of its emphasis on the person's learning to guide or instruct him-self or herself in a more effective manner. As in systematic de-sensitization, clients are asked to visualize a series of scenes along a continuum of increasing difficulty or anxiety and to imag-ine themselves responding to these situations. However, rather than the mastery-type imagery utilized in desensitization, a *cop-ing* imagery is emphasized. That is to say, the client is asked to imagine a scene in which anxiety and negative self-statements are usually experienced and is then guided by the therapist to substi-tute positive self-statements and relaxation procedures that will make the experience more manageable. The approach recognizes the reality of anxiety but utilizes guided practice, within the therapeutic session, to teach and strengthen coping responses. Homework assignments are given to practice this type of imagery repeatedly during the client's daily life.

Thus SIT can lead, as Meichenbaum (1975) points out, to clients' viewing anxiety "as positive and not debilitating (i.e., as a cue for employing their coping mechanisms)" (p. 375). Desensitization becomes, in Meichenbaum's words, an "active means of learning coping and self-control skills" (p. 375) rather than a passive procedure for counter-conditioning relaxed re-sponses. In addition, the positive human value of worrying is accepted but redirected into serving as a useful signal for the activation of coping responses. This is a more realistic goal with many clients than completely eliminating the tendency toward anxiety or worry. In effect, the client becomes reeducated: worry and tension are transformed into the normal cues needed to mobilize one's coping devices.

Modeling is similarly used in self-instructional training. The model is visualized in demonstrations of coping behaviors rather than of mastering a situation in an anxiety-free manner. Anxiety-lowering self-instructions, relaxation procedures, and the giving of self-reinforcement are included in each demonstration. Additionally, the model may show anxiety in the initial phases of the demonstration in order to increase the perceived similarity between model and the client observer.

Throughout the SIT process, whether desensitization procedures or modeling (followed by behavior rehearsal) is employed, there is a consistent emphasis on accepting and utilizing the client's learned pattern of worry and fear as a beginning point for change:

> ... the client's own maladaptive behavior is the cue, the reminder, to use the cognitive and behavioral techniques. In the past the client's symptoms were the occasion for worry, anxiety, depression and maladaptive behaviors, whereas following self-instructional training what the client says to himself about his symptoms has changed to a more adaptive way of functioning [Meichenbaum, 1975, p. 378].

Aspects of this approach were discussed in Chapter 8 in the section on stress management training. Yet another application can be seen in work with hyperactive children (Meichenbaum, 1979). A form of play therapy is utilized as the medium of the therapeutic encounter, but in contrast to the reflective and interpretive procedures of conventional play therapy, the clinician uses the session as an opportunity to reshape the child's self-dialogues. The therapist and child engage in various tasks during the play, and the therapist directly models the kind of guiding self-dialogue that can be used to contain frustration and expedite task accomplishment:

> Okay, what is it I have to do? You want me to copy the picture with the different lines. I have to go slowly and carefully. Okay, draw the lines down, good; then to the right, that's it; now down some more and to the left. Good, I'm doing fine so far. Remember, go slowly. Now back up again. No, I was supposed to go down. That's okay. Just erase the line carefully ... [Meichenbaum, 1979, p. 19].

Following modeling by the adult the child performs the task with overt guidance from the therapist. Further repetitions by the child encourage first spoken, then whispered self-instruction and, finally, covert self-guidance. The training procedure includes a series of tasks of increasing difficulty and complexity. Meichenbaum's (1979) review of self-control training with children summarizes the findings of a number of studies supporting on the effectiveness of this cognitively oriented approach. A recent controlled study (Kendall and Wilcox, 1980) found significant changes in social adjustment for the children receiving this cognitive approach. The gains were maintained at a one-month follow-up assessment.

Further Cognitive Change Techniques

Cognitively oriented procedures can be implemented at several levels or combined in a variety of ways with other helping interventions. Annon's (1976) PLISSIT model for brief therapy suggests that intervention should be attempted at the simplest possible level before turning to more complex procedures. The PLISSIT acronym stands for four potential levels of therapist activity, each of which may be complete in itself:

P = permission
LI = limited information
SS = specific suggestions
IT = intensive therapy

This model is a useful reminder that helping intervention need not be extensive or complex and for that reason alone is worth reviewing. Additionally the PLISSIT model will assist in articulating some of the varieties of cognitive intervention.

Permission (P). At this basic level the practitioner, as a socially sanctioned authority, offers the individual permission to act or feel in a certain way. For example, the vacillating parent is supported in taking a firm stance with an unruly adolescent. A key maneuver in Minuchin's (1978) work with anorectic adolescents and their families was to redefine the adolescent's refusal to eat as "rebelliousness" and to sanction the parents' taking a united stand against this behavior.

At a verbal level, moreover, the clinican can often effectively restructure detrimental beliefs and attitudes through minor intervention. In the chapter on behavior enactment this approach was illustrated in an account of a brief intervention designed to help hospitalized patients talk to their physicians about their medical condition. It was pointed out that it was helpful in the preparatory phases to shape certain of the patient's beliefs through such therapist statements as "You have a right to this information," "You have to take responsibility to get it," "You often have to teach your doctor how to talk to you," and so on. Therapist activity of this sort constitutes a type of cognitive restructuring—in effect a mild exhortation designed to counter some of the more common beliefs that can impede patient activiety or a redefinition ("You have to teach your doctor . . . ") designed to increase confidence.

At this level the clinician does not attempt to explore the client's belief system in any depth, but simply assumes that if the person is having difficulty in a given area of life, then it is likely that some of the more common human trepidations will be affecting functioning. Thus people who need to act assertively are troubled by notions of what others may think of them, parents struggle with high expectations of themselves or worry about the consequences of taking a firm stand with their chilren, sexual taboos inhibit freer communication or detract from the enjoyment of intimacy, and so on. None of these factors depends upon a highly refined "diagnostic" assessment on the clinician's part so much as on an imaginative and empathic knowledge of the human condition—what Schulman (1979) has called "preparatory empathy." Similarly, the individual client scarcely needs to "work through" these common roadblocks in some elaborate therapeutic process. For many people it is enough to have the clinician point out how prevalent such beliefs are and directly or indirectly give permission to discard or surmount them.

Limited information (LI). If necessary, the therapist can offer the client factual information on some key aspect of the problem. For example, people with medical difficulties are frequently able to manage the accompanying stress if knowledge of the extent or prognosis of their condition is made available to them.

I do not believe that we have paid enough attention to how providing accurate and timely information to a client constitutes a potent method of cognitive change. Some of the attitudes and beliefs that individuals hold are undoubtedly based on early experiences in their families of origin or may be characteristic of the overall social or cultural milieu in which they were reared. At the same time, there are some beliefs and attitudes that are based on a *lack* of information or knowledge in a particular area of life or on faulty information. Masters and Johnson (1970) identify the lack of accurate information about human sexuality as one of the major contributors to sexual dysfunction. Such beliefs as "Women have a lower sexual drive than men," "Masturbation can have detrimental physical effects," and "Older people have no interest in sex" are all untrue, yet are held by many people. Masters and Johnson bluntly characterize the source of these beliefs as "ignorance," and a significant component of their sexual therapy approach is devoted to the necessary reeducation.

Sexuality, of course, is a particularly troublesome area. Considering the lack of sexual education provided to most people and the general taboo against open discussion of sexual matters, it is not surprising to find widespread misinformation. Yet there can be significant gaps in other life areas which can act in a similar manner to promote or perpetuate human difficulty. Many young parents, for example, lack information on child-rearing practices and normal childhood development. Some honestly expect that a child should be fully toilet-trained by twelve months; some have little or no appreciation of the important developmental differences between girls and boys. Others have only scant knowledge about the expectations and demands of such intimate relationships as marriage.

Misinformation and myth are especially apparent in the areas of physical and mental health. People can become greatly alarmed at the somatic or emotional manifestations they may experience when dysfunction arises in either of these areas. A

case report drawn from Stein et al. (1971) illustrates this
phenomenon:

> A fifty-year-old man was seen for six sessions of brief therapy
> because of extreme nervousness and inability to work following a
> heart attack. Early sessions concentrated on exploration of the
> man's understanding of the physical damage the infarction had
> done and his misconceptions about these effects. Information on
> the working of the heart and the circulatory system was provided
> as his misunderstanding of this process was greatly increasing his
> anxiety about his physical status and ability to function.

In the emotional area Burns and Beck (1978), as Chapter 7
noted, point out how depressed individuals can regard their pessimistic thoughts and beliefs with the utmost seriousness. They
thus become locked into an insidious cycle of dysfunctional emotion based fundamentally on a lack of access to essential information. Earlier discussion in this chapter suggested how the cognitive therapist can provide the individual with authoritative information on this phenomenon. As I also noted, another method is to
orient the use of a daily diary toward the observation of the
pervasive thoughts or intruding beliefs that are affecting the
individual. In this strategy, instead of the therapist's supplying
information of a substantive or normative nature, clients gather
information on themselves, and this is incorporated into the
change process. The immediate objective is to make the client
more aware of these intrusions and, through this increased level
of knowledge, develop better control over their effects. One
might refer to this as "insight," but such an expansive term
seems inappropriate to the simple but significant change this type
of monitoring can induce. The therapist might *choose* to call it
"insight" if it appeared that such an explanation would appeal to
a particular client, but this would be a therapeutic maneuver
rather than a necessary consideration.

Specific suggestions (SS). At this level the client can be given
some specific directions to manage the problem. This can range
from brief instruction in relaxation methods to directions on how

to tell a potential sexual partner about one's difficulties with impotence. In a clinical example a young man who was given such directions was able to enter a new relationship without excessive anxiety. This in turn enabled him and his new partner to return for more extended counseling for his erectile problems.

Two particular cognitive change strategies, thought stopping and cognitive rehearsal, are worth discussing in more detail. For some individuals obsessive ruminative thoughts may be arousing dysfunctional levels of anxiety or interfering with important activities. Wolpe's (1973) thought-stopping technique can be a useful intervention in such instances. This simple self-management procedure, usually combined with other change strategies rather than employed alone, offers the client a minor but helpful self-control device.

Thought stopping is introduced by the therapist after the need to control ruminative thoughts has been clearly established. It is rehearsed in the therapeutic session, prior to any application in real life. The helper instructs the client to consciously begin the cycle of intruding thought and to signal when this is clearly present. At that moment the therapist shouts "Stop" to the client and then inquires about the effect of this sudden intrusion. Almost always the client, after he or she has recovered, will report at least a momentary interruption in the ruminative cycle, and the clinician used this as an opportunity to discuss the possibility of gaining further control. The sequence is rehearsed several more times within the session, with the client gradually taking over responsibility to say "Stop" at the appropriate moment. It can be helpful to have the client reinforce the use of the "Stop" signal by visualizing a pleasant scene or by verbalizing positive reinforcement. During these rehearsals the "Stop" signal is changed from a spoken to a subvocal form and the client is instructed to practice this covert version at home. Five to ten daily repetitions are advised, and after perhaps a week or two of practice the client is asked to use the procedure when disturbing thoughts intrude in real life.

There are also instances when a cognitive version of behavior rehearsal can be used to stimulate change. Kazdin (1973, 1974) offers empirical evidence that this approach can alter anxiety reactions or enhance assertiveness, and its effectiveness with even severe phobic conditions has been demonstrated (Bandura et al., 1980). Theoretically, cognitive rehearsal is based on modeling principles but utilizes the individual's own mental images as the source of the modeling demonstration. Thus individuals contending with difficulties in some aspect of an interpersonal relationship are instructed to visualize an imaginary vignette in which this difficulty is adequately managed. In this scene they are to imagine themselves or another individual coping in a more functional way. Thus Mr. Faber (see Chapter 3) was asked to mentally rehearse a series of scenes in which he interacted with young women in a confident and assured manner. As in behavior enactments the elements of more adequate performance can be arranged along a logical or emotional hierarchy and rehearsed in their appropriate sequence.

In employing cognitive rehearsal, the practitioner should keep several basic principles in mind. Initially, the scene that the client mentally rehearses should be closely monitored by the clinician. The client should describe aloud the essentials of this scene, or the clinician should literally instruct the client in what to picture. In addition, as Meichenbaum (1975) suggests in relation to self-instructional training, it is usually beneficial to employ a coping rather than a mastery theme in the visualization. That is to say, the client should imagine himself meeting with realistic difficulty but overcoming this rather than dealing with the situation without any real problem. Finally, once a scene has been rehearsed within the session, the client can be given the daily homework task of practicing a specific number of repetitions. Daily practice will tend to reinforce the effect of the cognitive rehearsal in enhancing self-efficacy and consequently reducing detrimental affect or cognition.

Intensive therapy (IT). Finally, where the preceding levels of intervention are insufficient to the client's needs, formal short-term therapy may be offered and, as in the model suggested throughout this work, should have a clearly negotiated contract and explicit goals. In the sexual area, for example, Annon (1976) suggests that clients who have not benefited from previous intervention may be suitable for the twelve- to 15-session intervention using the Masters and Johnson sexual counseling procedures. Similarly, short-term cognitively oriented intervention utilizing any of the major change approaches described earlier in this chapter may be judged appropriate to achieving the desired goals of treatment. As I have already stressed, these change strategies do not have to constitute the sole intervention but can frequently be combined with other approaches to problem solving or skill building as long as the total package offers an effective impetus toward goal attainment.

Chapter 10

Short-Term Treatment: An Afterview

HURRY UP PLEASE ITS TIME
—T. S. Eliot, *The Waste Land*

Setting modest but attainable goals has been a pervading theme of this book, and in accord with this recognition of the limitations of human endeavor, I will attempt to utilize these final pages in a particular way. There will be no attempt to restate or summarize my presentation of a model for planned short-term treatment. Instead, I will try to discuss several issues particularly germane to short-term practice which I believe have been suggested but not fully considered in the previous presentation. Additionally, aspects of this discussion will point out certain sources to which the aspiring brief therapist can turn in order to augment the guidelines offered in this work.

The Directive Stance in Therapy

In the preceding chapters an often active and participant stance has been advocated for the short-term therapist. This approach to the therapeutic role may create certain philosophical or value dilemmas for some practitioners or at least a sense of cognitive

230

dissonance with the therapeutic stance commonly taught. Twenty years ago Jerome Frank (1961) suggested that psychotherapeutic approaches, broadly considered, adopt either an evocative or a directive stance in relation to therapist–client interaction and therapeutic goals. He pointed out that evocative therapies have dominated North American approaches and are characteristized by a number of common features:

> Evocative therapies, often inaccurately termed "permissive," try to create a situation that will evoke the full gamut of the patient's difficulties and capabilities, thereby enabling him not only to work out better solutions for the problems bringing him to treatment but also to gain greater maturity, spontaneity, and inner freedom, so that he becomes better equipped to deal with future stresses as well as current ones. . . . Evocative therapies case a wider net, exploring in detail current problems, past experiences, dreams, and fantasies. They may pay special attention to the patient's feelings toward the therapist, which are viewed as closely related to the therapeutic process [p. 148].

The less fashionable directive approaches emphasize different facets of the therapeutic experience:

> [Directive] approaches try directly to bring about changes in the patient's behavior which, it is believed, will overcome his symptoms or resolve the difficulties for which he sought treatment. . . . [They] focus on the patient's current adjustment problems and review his past only sufficiently to enable the therapist to reach an understanding of his present difficulties. . . . In keeping with differences in their goals and approaches, directive therapies tend to be briefer than evocative therapies [p. 148].

Following Frank's definitions there is no doubt that the brief therapist takes a directive stance toward the management of helping, not only in relation to the initial interview but through much of the course of intervention. The very notion that helping should be "managed" implies an active and planned participation on the part of the helper.

Whether it is possible to be completely nondirective is disputable. Haley (1976) argues that it is not. For example, if the helper makes *any decision* about how he will conduct himself in relation to the client and attempts to carry this out in the interview, he will have some effect upon the client and at least to this extent is directive. The silent therapist, who might represent the height of nondirectiveness, can have a considerable impact on the client, particularly if the client expected that the therapist would be more active. Similarly, the therapist who directly or indirectly expresses the view that it is entirely up to the client to make decisions and choices (perhaps a more realistic version of the nondirective stance) is exerting a major pressure upon the client who had hoped that the therapist would take some (or even all) of this responsibility.

However, it is just as difficult to be totally directive. If the therapist is at all influenced by the client, then to that extent she or he is not directive. As the helper at least must gain some inkling of the kind of difficulty the client is experiencing, control must be relinquished in order to gain this information. To the extent that the helper allows the client to explicate his situation and is affected by that description, to that extent the helper is moving away from a radically directive stance.

Thus it is apparent that the notions of "directiveness" and nondirectiveness" are stereotypes rather than accurate pictures of therapeutic activity. The needs and expectations of the client influence the role of the helper in a variety of ways and cannot be separated from the activities of therapy. What might appear to be a relatively unstructured role with one client will appear highly directive in relation to another. In addition, just as it appears to be impossible to be completely nondirective, that is to say, to have no direct impact on the client, it is as unlikely that one can be completely directive and achieve complete control.

However, despite these general distinctions, I believe that the short-term counselor does take a more directive role within the helping relationship than therapists have generally been taught to do.

1. The helper takes considerable responsibility for conducting

the interview by such devices as asking questions to elicit needed information, limiting discussion in areas that do not appear to be immediately relevant, moving into areas of inquiry that do appear to be pertinent, and, in general, playing an assertive role in the immediate relationship.

2. Furthermore, the therapist takes responsibility for devising a plan of action that he or she believes will enable the client to resolve the problems being experienced. This strategy for change is explicitly discussed with the client so that he or she or will become aware of its nature and the demands it will exert, but developing the therapeutic plan is seen as the sole prerogative of the therapist.

3. Finally, the therapist assumes that the purpose of the helping encounter is to bring about beneficial and tangible change in the client, in line with the goals that have been mutually contracted. Unless there is *clear* reason to negate this contract, the practitioner utilizes the full range of therapeutic skills at his or her command toward achieving these goals.

Thus, underlying the directive approach to helping is a belief that therapy should have *directionality;* that is to say, it should be purposeful and goal-oriented. It will often be quite apparent, from the beginning of helping, that the couselor is taking such a stance. However, there may also be points in the treatment process when it is both useful and necessary to make this viewpoint clear. This may occur at a beginning point of helping with a client who, for example, has had several previously unsuccessful experiences with therapy. On the other hand, the assumption of directionality may need to be explicated at a midpoint in treatment to a client who has become bogged down within the very process of change. This latter instance represents the essence of the technique of confrontation—facing the client with the therapist's expectation that progress is not only necessary but mandatory if the helping relationship is to have any viable reason to continue.*

*See Hammond et al. (1977) for a lucid discussion of confrontation techniques in clinical practice.

Helpers may hesitate to assume a directive stance on the grounds that this approach may seriously limit the client's right to determine the nature and course of her or his life. Social workers, perhaps more than any other helping professionals, have stressed the principle of self-determination, and have often worked with groups of people, such as the poor and the various ethnic and racial minorities, whose lives have already been considerably limited by the restrictions of society. This heritage has made it more difficult for social workers to comfortably adopt a stance that may seem to place limitations on individual freedom. Several points need to be emphasized, however, in relation to this apparent conflict between therapist directiveness and client self-determination.

First, as short-term treatment begins, it should be readily apparent that the major goals of the initial interview postulated in Chapter 3 can hardly be viewed as seriously limiting the client's freedom or opportunity. To the contrary, the emphasis on arousing hope, responding to troublesome emotions, and identifying major life problems is much more likely to increase the client's ability to act. By doing these things, the tendency of such a direct approach to helping will be to serve as a stimulus toward freedom.

Second, the very process of defining a problem in specific and concrete terms makes the possibility of deciding whether to deal with this problem much clearer. The contract between helper and client can then be openly negotiated and both participants will be in a better position to knowledgeably consent to its demands. The essence of contracting, of course, is the mutual consent of the individuals involved. The client is always at some degree of disadvantage in any process of contracting as it is the client who is suffering from the effects of whatever the problem might be. To the extent that the client experiences such pressures, his or her choice cannot be regarded as completely free. However, even where freedom is limited by such pressures it is still better to have the choice of acting or not acting clearly posed, and there may well be times, at the beginning of treatment or later, when the client will decide that the *status quo* is preferable to the uncertainties of any movement or change. At such a moment the helper has no choice other than to accept and, indeed, respect the client's judgment.

Finally, while it is possible for this emphasis on therapist activity to be abused and for the practitioner to usurp the client's prerogatives, so is it possible for an overly permissive role to be detrimental. The confused and anxious client may suffer if the therapist does not exercise a needed and legitimate expertise in helping to identify problems and goals. The overriding consideration in either instance is the helping professional's ethical concern for the client's welfare and benefit. This, of course, is neither theory nor technology and ultimately can be governed by neither.

What Is the "Real" Problem?

Throughout this book I have suggested, often quite emphatically, that the purpose of short-term treatment is to help people to cope successfully with their problems in living. In discussing the process and goals of the initial interview, it was further emphasized that the clinician must pay close and serious attention to the client's expression of these difficulties and that any detailed exploration should be limited to the problem or two the client views as most pressing.

A related issue that is sometimes troublesome to clinicians is often expressed as doubt about whether the client, in the rapid engagement process typical of time-limited therapy, is actually revealing the "real" problem. This question has philosophical, theoretical, and practical implications that are worth examining.

Philosophically, of course, there is no doubt that the brief therapist is committed to the view that solving the immediate problems in living that impel people to seek professional help is the major purpose of therapeutic intervention. Furthermore, the brief therapist regards the client as the primary source of such problem identification. Epstein (1980) states this position very clearly:

> Clients know what their target problems are. They may need help in stating them and understanding them. Some clients may understand them perfectly. Often the client's target problem seems to be at odds with the problem identified by a referral source or with a professional view of what the problem out to be . . . [p. 49].

From this viewpoint, no matter how the practitioner may conceptualize the client's difficulties in relation to their etiology or current mainenance, the therapeutic obligation, if intervention is undertaken, is to enable the client to achieve a reasonable resolution of these difficulties.

At a theoretical level, practitioners may disagree about the most efficient way of treating a particular problem, with differing theories tending to emphasize selected aspects of the behavioral, affective, and cognitive components of the human experience. The pluralistic framework presented in this book is an attempt to recognize the place of all three of these major elements in promoting dysfunction and in facilitating change. Yet the philosophical or value stance remains the same: clients have a right to have the problems they identify taken seriously, and intervention must be directed to these chosen goals of the client.

It must be recognized, however, that practical difficulties can arise in identifying problems. As Reid and Epstein (1972) point out, some clients may initially identify less important or less embarrassing difficulties in the beginning moments of their first encounter with a comparative stranger. This is a natural human reaction in such a situation, but it does not mean that the clinician should routinely treat the client's initial descriptions as unimportant or superficial. Many clients, in my own experience, will reveal quite serious difficulties early in the first session, and those who disclose lesser concerns need to have these difficulties considered with empathy and compassion. Otherwise they will have little realistic basis for trusting the clinician and, consequently, revealing concerns that cut closer to the bone.

Some of this may also be a function of practitioner attitude. For example, as I have gained personal comfort and confidence in working in the sexual area, my ability to inquire directly about my clients' sexual problems has significantly increased. At the same time I still hear practitioners speaking of clients who are "not ready," even after many sessions, to talk about sexual difficulties. Yet I can see no difference between these clients and the clients with whom I have discussed sexual problems in the first interview. The question of *who* is "not ready" may be asked, particularly in relation to talking about life areas that are highly emotional or subject to social taboo.

Finally, there is always the possibility that a particular client may consciously withhold the revelation of a serious difficulty because of shame, anxiety, or distrust. In some cases this could create an obvious gap in the client's problem presentation, and, during the detailed inquiry phase of the initial interview, the therapist might directly ask about this missing information or related area of difficulty. For example, a parent might concentrate upon difficulties with a child and at the same time neglect to mention (or even deny) a discernible martial conflict. Yet even direct inquiries may not bring about acknowledgment of the problem.

When clients take such a stance, in my opinion they are making a choice which, in the final analysis, only they are entitled to make. They have decided not to deal with a particular difficulty or refuse to recognize that it is a problem in their lives. The clinican, in turn, is confronted with a number of possible choices:

1. Are the problems the client has revealed sufficiently troublesome to her or him that it is worthwhile expending professional (and client) effort in working on them? If so, therapy should proceed.

2. Are there such *obvious* (not conjectured) difficulties in other life areas that problem work on the difficulties the client has

shared would be patently useless? In such cases it is the therapist's responsibility to point out such an impasse. If the client does not agree to work on the obvious difficulties, a helping contract may not be possible.

3. Helper and client may initiate treatment around the revealed difficulties only to have the "hidden" problem thwart efforts at problem solving. Again, confrontation around the impasse is called for, and if the client agrees to change focus, a new contact may be negotiated.

4. Finally, therapist and client may work relatively successfully on a lesser problem and reach a suitable termination and evaluation point. At this time the client may reveal the unacknowledged problem and a further contract may be negotiated. Even if this does not transpire, the therapist has offered the client a legitimate helping experience in the problem area where the client chose to struggle. In any case, the practitioner's therapeutic ambitions should not interfere with the client's right to effective helping, even if this is in a relatively minor area of life.

Mobilizing Natural Remedial Influences

At several points I have briefly emphasized the importance of natural remedial processes in the therapeutic endeavor and suggested that, wherever possible, professional helping should reinforce and encourage these factors. The research evidence that sizable changes can occur in *untreated* groups of clients (Barrett et al., 1978; Bergin and Lambert, 1978; Sloane et al., 1975) suggests that in those who do receive treatment, the intervention in many respects is simply augmenting the effects of this so-called "spontaneous" recovery process. It is a sad fact that in certain studies the treated clients would have been better off in the untreated group (Fischer, 1976). Intervention, in other words, may interfere with natural remediation.

Cohn's report (1979) on a nationwide study of the treatment of child abuse and neglect offers further data on the potency of nonformal helping. This large-scale study compared profession-ally administered individual and group counseling with a "lay service" model of treatment. It should be noted, however, that the lay service package was not entirely nonprofessional but "in-cluded case management carried out by a full-time trained worker [and] also included the services of a lay person... who was assigned to the client as a friend, support and social contact" (p. 516). This combination, then, has some distinct resemblance to the augmentation of professional service by natural helping re-sources that is advocated here.

The individual, group, and lay service approaches were im-plemented in eight demonstration projects across the nation, and the final outcome evaluations showed a consistent advantage in six of the eight projects for the lay service model (53 percent improvement) in comparison with either individual (39 percent improvement) or group services (38 percent improvement). In one treatment center the lay service model was equivalent to professional services, and in only one program was it inferior. Additionally, Cohn notes, the combination of professional case management and lay helping was markedly less expensive than exclusively professional services. Cohn concludes that "treat-ment programs must mesh the use of professionals and lay per-sons in providing services" (p. 519), a sentiment which this discussion hearily echoes.

This phenomenon is of great importance to the helping profes-sions but, perhaps for ideological reasons, has been largely ne-glected. There is little or no systematic research on the charac-teristics of the natural remedial process, some theoretical frameworks have even deprecated its validity ("Flight into health"), and the clinician is left with only the scantiest of guid-ance on how to tap this potentially powerful force.

Golan (1980) points out that there is a continuum of helping sources available within the community and that, as Gurin, Ver-off, and Feld's (1960) landmark study of mental health services demonstrated, most individuals will turn to these resources for help rather than to the trained professional. In other words, formal counseling by mental health professionals is sought by a distinct minority, and for many of these only as a last resort. Golan identifies four levels of nonformal helping:

1. Initially the person will rely upon his or her own personal resources.
2. Then the natural help available from family, friends or neighbors will be utilized.
3. Mutual or self-help groups such as Parents Anonymous, Alcoholics Anonymous, and Recovery Inc. form yet another level of assistance.
4. Finally, the nonformal help offered by such community caregivers as teachers, police officers, and pastors in the course of their other duties is frequently available.

The therapist's task is to devise ways of connecting the client with these resources or, in other instances, of augmenting their effects. Thus, at a number of points throughout the case illustrations in this book, the therapist attempted to stimulate activities on the part of the client that would tap potential aspects of the natural remediation process. Some of these efforts were very simple—encouraging an individual to discuss a facet of a problem with a respected community figure such as a clergyman, employing a "commonsense" solution (such as problem solving) to a life difficulty, or guiding the client in gaining needed knowledge through reading. Other strategies were more broadly gauged and included the instigative emphasis (Kanfer, 1979) on change taking place in the natural environment, the stress placed in many of the social skill training approaches on developing self-regulated behavior, and the overall viewpoint (which may well be directly conveyed to the client) that the natural networks are generally helpful. Whether it is given direct or indirect expression, the therapist's concern is to deemphasize the therapeutic situation and, by highlighting the client's existing strengths and available resources, to mobilize these beneficial influences.

All this suggests that a major entry point to "spontaneous" or naturally induced change lies in stimulating the client's interaction with the network of relationships available within the current environment (Stevenson, 1961). Conversely, the debilitating power of social isolation can be seen in brainwashing techniques where the victim's interpersonal supports are deliberately limited in order to increase his or her vulnerability to influence (Frank, 1961; Watson, 1978). Natural remediation importantly involves mobilizing the available social forces, but difficulties can arise from both client and helper perspectives. On the one hand, clients may perceive their immediate friends and relatives as insensitive and uncaring and may hesitate to increase their interaction here. On the other hand, practitioners can become too absorbed in the minutiae of the therapeutic process and consequently may neglect the client's very real life outside these confines. Yet increased sharing and interaction with relatives and friends can have at least two major effects on the client:

1. The opportunity to discuss difficulties can be cathartic, similar to the effects seen within the therapeutic session, as the person is able to release pent-up emotion. The significant others can be supportive of the client and, in contrast to the therapist, are available on a continuous and permanent basis. In addition, the increased openness with close associates tends to promote the use of a resource that may prove useful in dealing with future problems. The client thus can obtain some immediate relief and, beyond this, learn a positive way of handling life difficulties.

Obviously there will be situations in which it is apparent that some of the people in the network are not able to offer this kind of support. Certain friends and relatives may be highly negative or even destructive in their attitudes and actions toward the client. Finally, some clients have depleted the resources of their social networks prior to turning to professional help, in what Langsley and Kaplan (1968) have characterized as the "Caretaker Crisis." (Even here, the objective of their short-term family therapy was not to offer a therapeutic haven to the distressed individual, but to restore the depleted social bonds that had previously maintained the client.)

Despite these potential drawbacks the therapist should not discount the help available from the client's natural social network even under apparently adverse circumstances. Furthermore, evaluating the helpfulness of the client's significant others should allow for a broad and flexible definition of helpfulness. Talking with a friend or relative is not going to be the same as talking to a therapist. Indeed, there is empirical evidence (Strong, 1971) that what people expect from a friend in times of trouble is sympathy and direct advice—not the more refined skills of the professional helper.

Finally, the clinician must remember that the client's existing network is the people with whom the client must continue to live. Not encouraging such contacts (or, worse still, discouraging them) can be a disservice to the client and can promote undue and unrealistic dependence on the therapist or the therapeutic setting. Some clients may need help in utilizing their natural resources, and assertion training or work on clearer communication is often useful in such cases. But the therapeutic effort, especially in short-term intervention, should heavily emphasize consistent utilization of the existing social network.

2. Aside from questions of social and emotional support, the client's increased sharing with immediate family and friends can have other beneficial effects. Often it is helpful to encourage clients to disclose to significant others their attempts to change themselves in important aspects of their lives. In other words, clients should make their efforts to handle a target problem public knowledge to some or even all of their associates. Disclosure of this kind can positively increase the client's commitment to change as it is transformed from a "secret" desire to an open stance.

A similar dynamic can be seen in the group modes of therapeutic intervention, and clients often refer, at least retrospectively, to this aspect of the group process. Self-help organizations such as Alcoholics Anonymous utilize variants of the same process. The very act of joining a self-help group is at least a semipublic recognition of difficulty. More specifically, AA encourages members in such acts of disclosure as openly acknowledging their alcoholism and, as one of the "Twelve Steps," "making amends" with neglected or injured friends and relatives. The moderate self-disclosure of one's efforts to change suggested here is an attempt to adapt this aspect of the natural remediation process to the context of individual helping.

Helping professionals sometimes react to this approach as contravening the principles of confidentiality and self-determination, but neither of these tenets need be violated. The clinician simply *suggests* a moderate degree of self-disclosure, with selected associates, and explains its potential benefits to the client. The client decides whether or not to share the relevant information, with whom, and to what extent. As in any therapeutic strategy it is the client, both immediately and ultimately, who decides the degree of participation. Similarly, it is the client who decides what amount of disclosure takes place and thereby places his or her own boundaries upon confidentiality.

Evaluating Treatment Outcome

The norms of clinical practice have paid scant heed to the issue of treatment effectivness. Clinicians are uneasy in the presence of researchers, and on their part, researchers find that they often have little to say to the front-line practitioner that is of any immediate practical value. Thus practitioners continue to rely on their own subjective judgment or the pronouncements of authoritative figures in the field; researchers seek grants, conduct studies, and publish reports which are read mostly by other researchers. This continuing schism results in helpers' not receiving vital information that could significantly strengthen their practice efforts. In addition, practice has suffered from its neglect of outcome evaluation through individual clinicians' not being encouraged to build this critical norm into their ongoing practice. In this latter sense, objective outcome evaluation becomes not only a part of responsible practice but a potentially valuable source of personal feedback for every clinician.

A major theme of this work has been the necessity of drawing upon and utilizing the findings of the psychotherapy research literature. The major theoretical frameworks have been placed in a secondary position to these empirically grounded generalizations. I do not believe, however, that every clinician should be a researcher. This appears to me to be as wrong-headed a view as the position, conveyed in some works, that every practitioner should be a consummate theoretician. Clinical practice is neither research nor theory, but the active application of certain contributions from each of these areas in the service of unhappy, troubled, and conflicted people. Clinicians need a good deal of help in this difficult work but cannot be expected to meet the requirements of either theory construction or research methodology.

Thus one cannot expect the front-line practitioner to evaluate treatment outcome in a manner that would meet the standards of a research study. Although outcome evaluation has much to offer to the practicing clinician, its demands must be scaled down and shaped to meet the realities of daily practice. Implicit in the model of brief treatment are some ways of achieving a suitable compromise between methodological rigor and practice reality.

For example, the efforts of the brief therapist to negotiate clear goals or objectives with the client around one or two major problems often make the need for elaborate evaluation devices unnecessary. It should be quite apparent at termination or follow-up whether the goals of intervention have been achieved. Short-term treatment's frequent concentration on immediate, practical objectives concerned with current living should similarly assist in evaluating the outcome of service. Has the client found a job? Has the move to a new apartment taken place? Is the client now able to obtain dates with women? These questions should be readily answerable from observation or discussion with the client. Although much of this information relies on self-reports from the client, the fact that brief treatment obtains such as assessment after a suitable follow-up interval will have some effect in reducing undue biasing effects.

However, there are times when more intangible effects must be measured or where client report and clinical judgment need corroboration. A series of clinically oriented scales have been developed by Walter Hudson (1977, in press) of the State University of Florida at Tallahassee which offer a highly useful tool in this task. The Hudson Scales have been explicitly designed for the exigencies of clinical practice and measure client status in five major areas that constitute frequent goals of clinical intervention:

1. Depression
2. Self-esteem
3. Marital Adjustment
4. Sexual adjustment
5. Parent-child relationships

Each scale is relatively short (twenty-five items) and can be completed by the typical client in five or ten minutes. The results can be immediately graded by the clinician and a score, ranging from 0 to 100, calculated. For each scale, Hudson's validation work suggests a clinical cutting point of 30—that is to say, any score between 30 and 100 represents clinically significant degrees of difficulty within the given area. As Hudson (1977) points out, this clinical cutting score provides an objective diagnostic criterion and also a means of judging the effectiveness of treatment. Additionally, this feature makes the results of any scale easily comprehensible to both clinician and client, and the scales are quite sensitive to the changes sought in treatment. I have found most clients quite willing to use these measures and, as might be expected, highly interested in the results. Hudson's discussion in his paper "A Measurement Package for Clinical Workers" (1977) offers many suggestions on their adaptation to practice, as well as complete versions of each scale.*

---

*Even more accessible versions of the Hudson Scales will be found in Fischer's *Effective Casework Practice: An Eclectic Approach* (1978) or in a forthcoming volume on social work research edited by Grinell (in press). The clinician is urged to experiment with the employment of these highly useful evaluative measures.

Follow-up Interviews: Issues and Benefits

Closely related to the issue of ongoing outcome assessment is the consistent employment of follow-up interviews as an integral part of clinical practice. The model of short-term treatment presented in this book has placed considerable emphasis on the need for a follow-up interview with every client. This interview is initiated by the therapist and is usually scheduled two to six months after the termination of the intervention. Unfortunately, most clinicans never see their clients following active treatment unless the client returns to seek further help. Yet systematic follow-up can provide important benefits to both clients and clinicians.

I noted briefly in an earlier chapter that there is some suggestive empirical evidence (Liberman, 1978) that in conjunction with an active, task-oriented approach, significant gains can take place following the actual cessation of intervention. Building in the routine employment of follow-up contact allows for the encouragement of such gains, and from a client perspective is a needed safeguard following any type of intervention—whether brief of lengthy, limited in focus or wide-ranging in scope. Has the client made meaningful gains that can endure past the immediate influence of the therapist-client relationship?

The client should be aware of the follow-up interview at an early stage of intervention. Mention of this practice can be included in the therapist's initial explanation of treatment, and it is helpful if, from time to time during intervention, the client is reminded that follow-up will occur at a specified interval following termination. This will make it clear that the follow-up session is not an intrusion into the client's private life or undertaken merely to satisfy the helper's curiosity, but is an integral part of the helping process. I do not attempt to set a specific date for the follow-up interview but usually indicate to the client that I will be in touch after a designated interval to arrange this session. The time preceding this contact should be clarified as offering the client an opportunity to test out and integrate the learning or change that has taken place during intervention.

In order to maintain a positive expectation about this process the follow-up session is characterized as "a chance to check on your progress" rather than an opportunity to determine whether the client's problems have returned. Similarly, a therapist may want to allow clients the freedom to initiate an interview prior to the actual follow-up session, but what is said about this too should be positively phrased. Thus my preference is to say, "Call me if you have any questions," rather than the more negative "Call me if you have any problems." The essential message concerning the clinician's availability is clear but does not create needless anticipation of difficulty.

Maluccio (1979) provides a fascinating account of a series of follow-up interviews with clients seen at a family service agency. He also interviewed the practitioners who had seen these clients and in some cases found an almost alarming discrepancy between the client's evaluation of service and the helper's perceptions. Generally the clients were highly positive about the help they had received, and they tended to evaluate this in terms of enhanced relationships, better job functioning, improved emotional and social life, and so on. The clinicans, none of whom apparently conducted follow-up interviews as part of their practice, were often still concerned about the conflicted or depleted state in which the client had entered treatment, and their judgments were biased by this more gloomy recollection. Without the salutory effect of hearing the client's realistic evaluation of improved functioning through follow-up contact, the practitioners were unable to appreciate either the tangible gains or the realistic limitations of their work.

A further benefit for the practitioner lies in the informative feedback the follow-up session can provide concerning the impact of various therapeutic techniques. It is extremely useful during the follow-up to ask the client specifically to evaluate the procedures used during intervention. What was most helpful? What aspects of therapy were not beneficial? What was gained from any aspect of treatment that can continue to be utilized in life? The therapist should emphasize that this sort of evaluation is an integral part of his or her own professional growth. Some clients can give only a very general assessment of treatment procedures, but on occasion, client feedback can be highly illuminating.

A thirty-two-year-old school teacher had been seen in a time-limited series of sessions which had focused on her difficulty in handling a lingering depression, related to unresolved grief around the death of her father. In a follow-up interview one year after termination she reported that her emotional and social functioning was quite satisfactory.

When asked to evaluate treatment, she identified an interview in which the therapist had utilized an experiential enactment technique as having been particularly helpful. The practitioner also thought that this procedure had been a turning point and saw the enactment (a variant of the "empty chair" technique) as forcing the client to recontact and face the submerged and evaded emotions which were preventing her from resolving her feelings about the deceased parent. The client, on the other hand, identified *the therapist's supportiveness* during the enactment as the most meaningful element in enabling her to cope with her grief.

Other clients may not be so dramatic in their recollections but can still provide the practitioner with an important source of feedback on treatment strategy. Along with this, of course, there is opportunity within the follow-up interview to negotiate a further helping contract if this proves necessary. Although the outcome studies of brief intervention are generally encouraging, there will be those who need (or want) further help. Follow-up interviews provide the client with this needed safeguard.

The Agency Setting: Constraints and Benefits

Most practitioners function within some sort of organizational structure, and, directly or indirectly, the characteristics of this setting affect the type and quality of therapeutic service offered.

Turner (1978) offers a cogent analysis of the many characteristics of formal organizations that can influence or mediate the effects of clinical practice. Initially he notes that "the very existence of agencies where some form of help or service is available manifests a form of social commitment" (p. 172) and this in turn confers legitimacy and authority upon the activities of the clinical practitioner. In other words, practitioners derive important supports for their professional activities from the organizational setting, as well as from their professional status.

He also considers the broad question of *accessibility* of service and suggests that three component aspects of this issue must be critically examined—physical location, time elements, and client perception. Advocates of short-term treatment have been strongly influenced by their perception of a need for more efficient services, and this corollary issue of accessibility merits further discussion.

There is certainly some trend for agencies and clinics in the human services to set up neighborhood centers or outreach offices in order to offer easier access to clients. There is no doubt that reducing client travel time, for instance, or increasing the agency's perceived identification with the neighborhood can have important positive effects. The findings from military crisis intervention (Watson, 1978) suggest yet another benefit in this trend—clients in emotional turmoil may feel less alienated and disconnected from their natural support systems if intervention is conducted as close as possible to these familiar surroundings. Perhaps the logical extension of this argument would be the consistent utilization of interviews in the home, and indeed some have advocated this practice (Freidman et al., 1965). However, the realities of greatly expanded travel time for staff in an era of shrinking funding make any large-scale use of home-based interviews difficult, if not impossible. The use of outreach centers, wherever possible, along with a clear orientation toward the mobilization of the natural helping sources, appears to be a needed compromise.

Turner sees two related aspects to the time component in service accessibility: (1) How long must the client wait for service to begin? (2) During what hours are helping services actually available? Short-term treatment is directly aimed at alleviating lengthy waiting periods for service and reducing the trend toward unplanned drop-out that such waiting promotes. Leventhal and Weinberger's (1975) large-scale study of agency practice indicates that adopting a predominant mode of brief intervention does have these beneficial effects and yet continues to maintain an effective level of service.

Within what working hours service should be offered is a knottier question and one on which little if any objective data are available. One hears practitioners complain from time to time about the difficulties of involving fathers and husbands in treatment, but I have usually found, on further inquiry, that the agency concerned rarely stayed open after 5 P.M. My own experience in a family service agency open until 10 P.M. three nights a week has been exactly the opposite. This is not to say that every father and husband was easily involved or completely cooperative, but where ample evening hours are available, engagement is not a major problem. This consideration appears especially important where an agency hopes to offer service to working-class or low socioeconomic populations. Such clients often have little flexibility in their working hours and no option of taking time off without suffering direct loss of income.

Finally, Turner suggests that the perceived attributes of the agency may limit or enhance its accessibility. This is a complex factor that can involve anything from the name of the organization—does this suggest restriction to a particular client group or target problem?—to questions concerning its reputation in the community. Perhaps the most important aspect of an agency's reputation is not the view held by other professionals so much as its reputation among its clients, past and potential. Do these clients form a supporting network which, among other functions, refers new clients to the agency? Such a phenomenon not only can enhance effectiveness with the new clients but in some instances is a significant source of evaluative data on previous work.

Mr. and Mrs. Smithson were seen for six sessions of marital counseling but by the time of follow-up had decided to separate and divorce. The practitioner, like many marital therapists, was perplexed about the desirability of this outcome as it had not been an explicit goal of counseling. However, he was reassured somewhat later when Mr. and Mrs. Smithson referred two other couples for marriage counseling, thus indicating (at least indirectly) that the outcome had been satisfactory to them.

Many other aspects of organizational structure and functioning can impact upon therapeutic services. For instance, staff morale has been a concern of many administrators, and it is common knowledge that absenteeism, staff turnover, and general efficiency and productivity are affected by this broad variable. There are even more compelling reasons to pay close attention to clinician morale within a mental health setting. As review of the psychotherapy research literature (Frank, 1979; Garfield, 1980) suggests a major factor in therapeutic effectiveness lies in a number of personal qualities of the therapist as these are conveyed within the helping relationship. These qualities or skills—for instance, empathy, genuineness, assertiveness, or any number of complex interviewing and change techniques—cannot be regarded as simply technological factors. They are closely related to the personal well-being of the practitioner and, as I have commented in other writing (Wells, in press), must be carefully protected and nurtured by the administrator.

Administrators, in other words, must seriously examine their management procedures in respect to the question of staff morale. Are current procedures, whatever their convenience or efficiency, adversely affecting morale? Beyond this question the administrator must also ask what specific efforts, whether through improved working conditions, personal recognition, relief from excessive emotional stress, or the resources of consultation and supervision, can be mobilized to sustain the spirit of the front-line practitioner. If the therapist and the qualities this individual con-

veys are a key factor in effective outcome, what is the administrator doing to support this vital human equation?

To counterbalance this emphasis on what the administrator or
the organizational setting can give to the practitioner, it will also
be useful to examine how the practitioner can function more
effectively within the organization. Pruger (1978) examines this
issue in provocative terms. He suggests that it is both inaccurate
and misleading to place all of the responsibility for effective
organizational functioning on the shoulders of the administrator.
The individual practitioner, despite protestations about the awesome power of the organizational system, has much more scope
for self-direction and effective functioning within this system
than is generally acknowledged. Indeed, the individual's capacity
for at least relative autonomy is the central theme of Pruger's
intriguing analysis of bureaucratic functioning as an essential
practitioner skill.

He contends that both professional training and ideology leave
the practitioner poorly prepared to cope with organizational life.
Although almost all helping services are implemented through
organizations, large and small, there is scant recognition of the
need for ''explicit instruction to increase the practitioner's ability
to mitigate the stresses, avoid the traps, and develop the possibilities that inhere in the bureaucratic environment'' (p. 151).
Ideologically, moreover, professionally trained staff have contended that *they* are not bureaucrats; as Pruger pointedly remarks,
''the professional does everything the bureaucrat does, but still
resists any conception of himself or herself as a bureaucrat'' (p.
153).

The personal recognition of one's undeniable role within the
organizational system is the first step toward achieving more
effective functioning within this milieu. Beyond this, Pruger's
analysis suggests a number of ways in which the individual practitioner can gain (or lose) autonomy or, at other points, play a part
in inducing institutional change. For example, he points out that
the power of any bureaucracy is not all-ecompassing, but is more
in the nature of ''power to elicit on average certain predictable

responses to organizational situations'' (p. 158). The individual practitioner has a significant degree of discretion within this structure but must be careful not to heedlessly give it away through either ignorance or apathy. Although acknowledging that many of the skills for organizational functioning are still unspecified, Pruger offers an insightful analysis of how to increase one's awareness and facility. His paper, only sketchily reviewed here, should be mandatory reading for all practitioners.

A Final Note: Marital, Family, and Group Approaches

Although I have largely concentrated on the principles and techniques of one-to-one intervention in this work, there is no doubt that the time-limited approaches can be readily operationalized in marital, family, and group modalities of treatment. In this section I will identify a few key references in each area.

As in individual treatment, there is some research evidence that planned short-term therapy with marital couples and families is at least as effective as long-term intervention (Gurman and Kniskern, 1978; Wells, in press). Moreover, in Reid and Shyne's (1969) carefully designed study of short-term treatment the marital cases achieved significantly better outcome, a finding partially replicated by Wattie (1973). Although no definitive text has yet been written on short-term marital or family work, many of the articles in Gurman and Rice's (1975) *Couples in Conflict* and Olsen's (1976) more broadly focused *Treating Relationships* describe relatively brief, structured approaches. These many papers, along with the more detailed descriptions of clinical practice offered (from varying theoretical perspectives) by such authors as Ables and Brandsma (1977), Wells and Figurel (1979) and Jacobson and Margolin (1979), should provide a good introduction.

Time-limited group treatment has frequently concentrated on the development of specific social skills and within this context has been utilized with a wide range of client populations. However, brief group treatment has been employed in many other ways, and an annotated bibliography which I edited a few years ago (Wells, 1976) identifies references to a number of these applications. Beyond these sources, Garvin (1974) has written specifically on task-centered group approaches, Waxer (1977) discusses short-term group techniques, while Rose's (1977) book on behavioral group therapy describes several of the skill training approaches that can be adapted to group intervention. These will serve as an entry point into the literature although, like short-term marital and family therapy, brief group approaches deserve a more concentrated consideration than is currently available.

References

ABLES, B. S., AND BRANDSMA, J. M. *Therapy with Couples.* San Francisco: Jossey-Bass, 1977.

ALBERTI, R. E., AND EMMONS, M. L. *Your Perfect Right.* San Luis Obispo, CA: Impact, 1974.

ANNON, J. S. *Behavioral Treatment of Sexual Problems,* Vol. 1, *Brief Therapy.* New York: Harper & Row, 1976.

BACH, G. AND WYDEN, R. *The Intimate Enemy.* New York: Morrow, 1968.

BAEKLAND, F., AND LUNDWALL, L. Dropping out of treatment: A critical review. *Psychological Bulletin,* 1975, *82,* 738–783.

BAEKLAND, F., LUNDWALL, L., AND KISSIN, B. Methods for the treatment of chronic alcoholism: A critical appraisal. In R. J. Gibbins, Y. Israel, H. Kalant, R. E. Popham, W. Schmidt, and R. G. Smart (Eds.), *Research Advances in Alcohol and Drug Problems,* Vol. II. New York: Wiley, 1975.

BANDLER, R., AND GRINDER, J. *The Structure of Magic: A Book about Language and Therapy.* Palo Alto, CA: Science and Behavior Books, 1976.

BANDLER, R., GRINDER, J., AND SATIR, V. *Changing with Families,* Vol. 1. Palo Alto, CA: Science and Behavior Books, 1976.

BANDURA, A. *Principles of Behavior Modification.* New York: Holt, Rinehart and Winston, 1969.

BANDURA, A. Self-efficacy: Toward a unifying theory of behavioral change. *Psychological Review,* 1977a, *2,* 191–215.

BANDURA, A. *Social Learning Theory*. Englewood Cliffs, N.J.: Prentice Hall, 1977b.

BANDURA, A., ADAMS, N. E., HARDY, A. B., AND HOWELLS, G. N. Tests of the generality of self-efficacy theory. *Cognitive Therapy and Research*, 1980, *4*, 39–66.

BARBACH, L. G. Group treatment of pre-orgasmic women. *Journal of Sex and Marital Therapy*, 1974, *1*, 139–145.

BARBACH, L. G. *Women Discover Orgasm*. New York: Free Press, 1980.

BARRETT, C. L., HAMPE, I. E., AND MILLER, L. Research on psychotherapy with children. In S. L. Garfield and A. E. Bergin (Eds.), *Handbook of Psychotherapy and Behavior Change*, 2nd ed. New York: Wiley, 1978.

BARTEN, H. H. The coming of age of the brief psychotherapies. In L. Bellak and H. H. Barten (Eds.), *Progress in Community Mental Health*. New York: Grune & Stratton, 1969.

BARTEN, H. H. (Ed.) *Brief Therapies*. New York: Behavioral Publications, 1971.

BARTEN, H. H., AND BARTEN, S. S. (Eds.) *Children and Their Parents in Brief Therapy*. New York: Behavioral Publications, 1973.

BECK, A. T. *Cognitive Therapy and the Emotional Disorders*. New York: International Universities Press, 1976.

BECK, D. F. *Patterns in the Use of Family Agency Service*. New York: Family Service Association of America, 1962.

BECK, D. F. Research findings on the outcomes of marital counseling. *Social Casework*, 1975, *56*, 153–181.

BECK, D. F., AND JONES, M. A. *Progress on Family Problems*. New York: Family Service Association of America, 1973.

BEDNAR, R. L., AND LAWLIS, G. F. Empirical research in group psychotherapy. In A. E. Bergin and S. L. Garfield (Eds.), *Handbook of Psychotherapy and Behavior Change*, 1st ed. New York: Wiley, 1971.

BENSON, H. Your innate asset for combating stress. *Harvard Business Review*, 1974, *52*, 49–60.

BERGIN, A. E. The evaluation of therapeutic outcomes. In A. E. Bergin and S. L. Garfield (Eds.), *Handbook of Psychotherapy and Behavior Change*, 1st ed. New York: Wiley, 1971.

BERGIN, A. E., AND LAMBERT, M. J. The evaluation of therapeutic outcomes. In S. L. Garfield and A. E. Bergin (Eds.), *Handbook of Psychotherapy and Behavior Change,* 2nd ed. New York: Wiley, 1978.

BROWN, EMILY. Divorce counseling. In D. H. L. Olsen, *Treating Relationships.* Lake Mills, IA: Graphic Press, 1976.

BURGOYNE, R. W., STAPLES, F. R., YAMAMOTO, J., WOLKON, G. H., AND KLINE, F. Patients' requests of an outpatient clinic. *Archives of General Psychiatry,* 1979, *36,* 400–403.

BURNS, D. D., AND BECK, A. T. Cognitive behavior modification of mood disorders. In J. P. Foreyt and D. P. Rathjen (Eds.), *Cognitive Behavior Therapy.* New York: Plenum, 1978.

BUTCHER, J. N., AND KOSS, M. P. Research on brief and crisis-oriented therapies. In S. L. Garfield and A. E. Bergin (Eds.), *Handbook of Psychotherapy and Behavior Change,* 2nd ed. New York: Wiley, 1978.

CAPLAN, G. *Principles of Preventive Psychiatry.* New York: Basic Books, 1964.

CARKHUFF, R. R. *Helping and Human Relationships,* Vols. I and II. New York: Holt, Rinehart and Winston, 1969.

CHESNEY, M., AND SHELTON, J. L. A comparison of muscle relaxation and electromyogram biofeedback treatments for muscle contraction headaches. *Journal of Behavior Therapy and Experimental Psychiatry,* 1976, *7,* 221–226.

COHN, A. H. Effective treatment of child abuse and neglect. *Social Work,* 1979, *24,* 513–519.

CORSINI, R. J. *Roleplaying in Psychotherapy.* Chicago: Aldine, 1966.

DAVENLOO, H. (Ed.) *Basic Principles and Techniques of Short-Term Dynamic Psychotherapy.* New York: SP Medical and Scientific Books, 1978.

DILORETO, A. O. *Comparative Psychotherapy: An Experimental Analysis.* Chicago: Aldine-Atherton, 1971.

DOLEYS, D. M. Behavioral treatments for nocturnal enuresis in children: A review of the recent literature. *Psychological Bulletin,* 1977, *44,* 31–54.

DUNLAP, K. *Habits: Their Making and Unmaking.* New York: Liveright, 1932.

D'ZURILLA, T. J., AND GOLDFRIED, M. R. Problem-solving and behavior modification. *Journal of Abnormal Psychology,* 1971, *78,* 107–126.

ELLIS, A. *Reason and Emotion in Psychotherapy.* New York: Lyle Stuart, 1962.

ELLIS, A. *Growth Through Reason.* North Hollywood, CA: Wilshire, 1971.

EPSTEIN, L. *Helping People: The Task-centered Approach.* St. Louis: Mosby, 1980.

ERIKSON, E. H. *Childhood and Society.* New York: Norton, 1950.

EWING, C. P. *Crisis Intervention as Psychotherapy.* New York: Oxford University Press, 1978.

EYSENCK, H. J. The effects of psychotherapy: An evaluation. *Journal of Consulting Psychology,* 1952, *16,* 319–324.

FENSTERHEIM, H., AND BAER, J. *Don't Say Yes When You Want to Say No.* New York: McKay, 1975.

FISCHER, J. *The Effectiveness of Social Casework.* Springfield, IL: Thomas, 1976.

FISCHER, J. *Effective Casework Practice: An Eclectic Approach.* New York: McGray-Hill, 1978.

FORD, D. H., AND URBAN, H. B. *Systems of Psychotherapy: A Comparative Analysis.* New York: Wiley, 1963.

FRANK, J. D. *Persuasion and Healing,* 1st ed. Baltimore: Johns Hopkins University Press, 1961.

FRANK, J. D. The role of hope in psychotherapy. *International Journal of Psychiatry,* 1968, *5,* 383–395.

FRANK, J. D. Common features account for effectiveness. *International Journal of Psychiatry,* 1969, *7,* 122–127.

FRANK, J. D. Expectation and therapeutic outcome: The placebo effect and the role induction interview. In J. D. Frank, R. Hoehn-Saric, S. D. Imber, B. L. Liberman, and A. R. Stone (Eds.), *Effective Ingredients of Successful Psychotherapy.* New York: Brunner/Mazel, 1978.

FRANK, J. D. The present status of outcome studies. *Journal of Consulting and Clinical Psychology,* 1979, *47,* 310–316.

FREIDMAN, A. S., BOSZORMENYI-NAGY, I., JUNGREIS, J., LINCOLN,

References   259

G., MITCHELL, H. E., SONNE, J. C., SPECK, R., AND SPIVAK, G. *Psychotherapy for the Whole Family.* New York: Springer, 1965.

FREUD, A. *The Ego and Mechanisms of Defense.* New York: International Universities Press, 1946.

GALASSI, J. P., AND GALASSI, M. D. Modification of heterosocial skill deficits. In A. S. Bellack and M. Hersen (Eds.), *Research and Practice in Social Skills Training.* New York: Plenum, 1978.

GARFIELD, S. L. Research on client variables in psychotherapy. In A. E. Bergin and S. L. Garfield (Eds.), *Handbook of Psychotherapy and Behavior Change,* 1st ed. New York: Wiley, 1971.

GARFIELD, S. L. Basic ingredients or common factors in psychotherapy? *Journal of Consulting and Clinical Psychology,* 1973, *41,* 9–12.

GARFIELD, S. L. *Psychotherapy: An Eclectic View.* New York: Wiley, 1980.

GARFIELD, S. L., AND KURTZ, R. A study of eclectic views. *Journal of Consulting and Clinical Psychology,* 1977, *45,* 78–83.

GARVIN, C. Task-centered groupwork. *Social Service Review,* 1974, *48,* 494–507.

GIBBONS, J. S., BOW, I., BUTLER, J., AND POWELL, J. Client's reactions to task-centered casework: A follow-up study. *British Journal of Social Work,* 1979, *9,* 203–215.

GITTELLMAN, M. Behavior rehearsal as a technique in child treatment. *Journal of Child Psychology and Psychiatry,* 1965, *6,* 251–255.

GOLAN, N. Crisis theory. In F. J. Turner (Ed.), *Social Work Treatment: Interlocking Theoretical Approaches.* New York: Free Press, 1974.

GOLAN, N. *Treatment in Crisis Situations.* New York: Free Press, 1978.

GOLAN, N. Intervention at times of transition: Sources and forms of help. *Social Casework,* 1980, *61,* 259–266.

GOLDFRIED, M. R., AND DAVISON, G. C. *Clinical Behavior Therapy.* New York: Holt, Rinehart and Winston, 1976.

GOLDFRIED, M. R., AND GOLDFRIED, A. P. Cognitive change methods. In F. H. Kanfer and A. P. Goldstein (Eds.), *Helping People Change.* New York: Pergamon, 1975.

GOLDSTEIN, M. J., RODNICK, E. H., EVANS, J. R., MAY, P. R. A.,

AND STEINBERG, M. R. Drug and family therapy in the aftercare of acute schizophrenics. *Archives of General Psychiatry,* 1978, *35,* 1169–1177.

GREENE, M. Some recent contributions to a noneclectic approach. *Clinical Social Work Journal,* 1978, *6,* 171–187.

GRIER, W. H., AND COBBS, F. R. *Black Rage.* New York: Basic Books, 1968.

GRINELL, R. M., JR. (Ed.), *Social Work Research and Evaluation.* Itasca, IL: F. E. Peacock, in press.

GUERNEY, B. G. *Relationship Enhancement: Skill-Training Programs for Therapy, Problem Prevention and Enrichment.* San Francisco: Jossey-Bass, 1977.

GUERNEY, B. G., STOLLAK, G., AND GUERNEY, L. The practicing psychologist as educator: An alternative to the medical practitioner model. *Professional Psychology,* 1971, *2,* 276–282.

GURIN, G., VEROFF, J., AND FELD, S. *Americans View Their Mental Health.* New York: Basic Books, 1960.

GURMAN, A. S. Some therapeutic implications of marital therapy research. In A. S. Gurman and D. G. Rice (Eds.), *Couples in Conflict: New Directions in Marital Therapy.* New York: Aronson, 1975.

GURMAN, A. S., AND KNISKERN, D. Research in marital and family therapy: Progress, perspective, and prospect. In S. L. Garfield and A. E. Bergin (Eds.), *Handbook of Psychotherapy and Behavior Change,* 2nd ed. New York: Wiley, 1978.

GURMAN, A. S., AND RAZIN, A. M. (Eds.) *Effective Psychotherapy: A Handbook of Research.* New York: Pergamon, 1977.

GURMAN, A. S., AND RICE, D. G. *Couples in Conflict: New Directions in Marital Therapy.* New York: Aronson, 1975.

HALEY, J. *Strategies of Psychotherapy.* New York: Grune & Stratton, 1963.

HALEY, J. Commentary. In J. Haley (Ed.), *Advanced Techniques of Hypnosis and Therapy.* New York: Grune & Stratton, 1967.

HALEY, J. *Uncommon Therapy.* New York: Norton, 1974.

HALEY, J. *Problem-solving Therapy.* San Francisco: Jossev-Bass. 1976.

HAMMOND, J., HEPWORTH, D. H., AND SMITH, V. *Improving Therapeutic Communication.* San Francisco: Jossey-Bass, 1977.

HANSELL, N. *A Primer of Mental Health Advances*. Elgin, IL: New Orient Media, 1973 (six audiotape cassettes).

HANSELL, N. *The Person-in-Distress*. New York: Behavioral Publications, 1975.

HARTMANN, H. *Ego Psychology and the Problem of Adaptation*. New York: International Universities Press, 1958.

HATCHER, C., AND HIMELSTEIN, P. *The Handbook of Gestalt Therapy*. New York: Aronson, 1976.

HEPWORTH, D. H. Early removal of resistance in task-centered casework. *Social Work*, 1979, *24* 317–323.

HERZBERG, A. Short treatment of neurosis by graduated tasks. *British Journal of Medical Psychology*, 1941, *19*, 36–51.

HOLMES, T. H., AND RAHE, R. H. The social readjustment rating scale. *Journal of Psychosomatic Research*, 1967, *11*, 213–218.

HUDSON, W. W. A measurement package for clinical workers. Paper presented at the Council on Social Work Education 23rd Annual Program Meeting, Phoenix, AZ, February 1977.

HUDSON, W. W. Index and scale construction. In R. M. Grinell, Jr. (Ed.), *Social Work Research and Evaluation*. Itasca, IL: F. E. Peacock, in press.

JACKSON, D. D. (Ed.) *Communication, Family and Marriage*. Palo Alto, CA: Science and Behavior Books, 1965.

JACOBSON, E. *Progressive Relaxation*. Chicago: University of Chicago Press, 1929.

JACOBSON, G. Crisis theory and treatment strategy: Some sociocultural and psychodynamic considerations. *Journal of Nervous and Mental Disease*, 1965, *141*, 209–218.

JACOBSON, N. S., AND MARGOLIN, G. *Marital Therapy: Strategies Based on Social Learning and Behavior Exchange Principles*. New York: Brunner/Mazel, 1979.

JAKUBOWSKI-SPECTOR, P. Facilitating the growth of women through assertive training. *The Counseling Psychologist*, 1973, *4*, 75–86.

JAYARANTNE, S. A study of clinical eclecticism. *Social Service Review*, 1978, *52*, 621–631.

KANFER, F. H. Self-managment: Strategies and tactics. In A. P. Goldstein and F. H. Kanfer (Eds.), *Maximizing Treatment Gains: Transfer Enhancement in Psychotherapy*. New York: Academic Press, 1979.

262   REFERENCES

KANFER, F. H., AND GOLDSTEIN, A. P. *Helping People Change.* New York: Pergamon, 1975.

KAZDIN, A. E. Covert modeling and the reduction of avoidance behavior. *Journal of Abnormal Psychology,* 1973, *81,* 87–95.

KAZDIN, A. E. Effects of covert modeling and model reinforcement on assertive behavior. *Journal of Abnormal Psychology,* 1974, *83,* 240–252.

KAZDIN, A. E. Sociopsychological factors in psychopathology. In A. S. Bellack and M. Hersen (Eds.), *Research and Practice in Social Skills Training.* New York: Plenum, 1978.

KAZDIN, A. E., AND WILSON, G. T. *Evaluation of Behavior Therapy: Issues, Evidence and Research Strategies.* Cambridge, MA: Ballinger, 1978.

KEILSON, M. V., DWORKIN, F. H., AND GELSO, C. J. The effectiveness of time-limited psychotherapy in a university counseling center. *Journal of Clinical Psychology,* 1979, *35,* 631–636.

KENDALL, P. C., AND WILCOX, L. E. Cognitive-behavioral treatment for impulsivity: Concrete versus conceptual training in non-self-controlled children. *Journal of Consulting and Clinical Psychology,* 1980, *48,* 80–91.

KOSS, M. P. Length of psychotherapy for clients seen in private practice. *Journal of Consulting and Clinical Psychology,* 1979, *47,* 210–212.

LANGE, A. J., AND JAKUBOWSKI, P. *Responsible Assertive Behavior: Cognitive/Behavioral Procedures.* Champaign, IL: Research Press, 1976.

LANGSLEY, D. G. Comparing clinic and private practice of psychiatry. *American Journal of Psychiatry,* 1978, *135,* 702–706.

LANGSLEY, D. G., AND KAPLAN, D. K. *The Treatment of Families in Crisis.* New York: Grune & Stratton, 1968.

LANGSLEY, D. G., MACHOTKA P., AND FLOMENHAFT, K. Avoiding mental hospital admission: A follow-up study. *American Journal of Psychiatry,* 1971, *127,* 1391–1394.

LANSKY, M. R., AND DAVENPORT, A. E. Difficulties in brief conjoint treatment of sexual dysfunction. *American Journal of Psychiatry,* 1975, *132,* 177–179.

LAZARE, A., COHEN, F., JACOBSON, A., WILLIAMS, R., MIGNONE, R.,

AND ZISOOK, S. The walk-in patient as a "customer": A key dimension in evaluation and treatment. *American Journal of Orthopsychiatry*, 1972, *42*, 872–883.

LAZARE, A., EISENTHAL, S., AND WASSERMAN, L. The customer approach to patienthood. *Archives of General Psychiatry*, 1975a, *32*, 553–558.

LAZARE, A., EISENTHAL, S., WASSERMAN, L., AND HARFORD, I. Patient requests in a walk-in clinic. *Comprehensive Psychiatry*, 1975b, *16*, 467–477.

LAZARUS, A. A., AND FAY, A. *I Can If I Want To*. New York: Morrow, 1975.

LENNARD, H. J., AND BERNSTEIN, A. *The Anatomy of Psychotherapy*. New York: Columbia University Press, 1960.

LEVENTHAL, T., AND WEINBERGER, G. Evaluation of a large-scale brief therapy program for chilren. *American Journal of Orthopsychiatry*, 1975, *49*, 119–133.

LEWIS, M. S., GOTTESMAN, D., AND GUTSTEIN, S. The course and duration of crisis. *Journal of Consulting and Clinical Psychology*, 1978, *47*, 128–134.

LIBERMAN, B. L. The role of mastery in psychotherapy: Maintenance of improvement and prescriptive change. In J. D. Frank, R. Hoehn-Saric, S. D. Imber, B. L. Liberman, and A. R. Stone (Eds.), *Effective Ingredients of Successful Psychotherapy*. New York: Brunner/Mazel, 1978.

LINEHAN, M. M., AND EGAN, K. J. Assertion training for women. In A. S. Bellack and M. Hersen (Eds.), *Research and Practice in Social Skills Training*. New York: Plenum, 1978.

LOPICCOLO, J., AND LOPICCOLO, L. *Handbook of Sex Therapy*. New York: Plenum, 1978.

LORION, R. P. Research on psychotherapy and behavior change with the disadvantaged. In S. L. Garfield and A. E. Bergin (Eds.), *Handbook of Psychotherapy and Behavior Change*, 2nd ed. New York: Wiley, 1978.

LUBORSKY, L., CHANDLER, M., AUERBACH, A. H., COHEN, J., AND BACHRACH, H. M. Factors influencing the outcome of psychotherapy. *Psychological Bulletin*, 1971, *75*, 145–185.

LUBORSKY, L., SINGER, B., AND LUBORSKY, L. Comparative studies of psychotherapies. *Archives of General Psychiatry,* 1975, *32,* 995–1008.

LUKTON, R. C. Crisis theory: Review and critique. *Social Service Review,* 1974, *48,* 384–402.

MCCARY, J. *Human Sexuality: A Brief Edition.* New York: Van Nostrand, 1973.

MCFALL, R. M., AND LILLIESAND, D. V. Behavior rehearsal with modeling and coaching in assertive training. *Journal of Abnormal Psychology,* 1971, *77,* 313–323.

MCFALL, R. M., AND TWENTYMAN, C. T. Four experiments on the relative contributions of rehearsal, modeling and coaching to assertion training. *Journal of Abnormal Psychology,* 1973, *81,* 199–218.

MAHONEY, M. J. *Cognition and Behavior Modification.* Cambridge, MA: Ballinger, 1974.

MAHONEY, M. J., AND ARKOFF, D. B. Cognitive and self-control therapies. In S. L. Garfield and A. E. Bergin (Eds.), *Handbook of Psychotherapy and Behavior Change,* 2nd ed. New York: Wiley, 1978.

MALUCCIO, A. *Learning from Clients.* New York: Free Press, 1979.

MANN, J. *Time-limited Psychotherapy.* Cambridge, MA: Harvard University Press, 1973.

MARKS, I. Behavioral psychotherapy with adult neurosis. In S. L. Garfield and A. E. Bergin (Eds.), *Handbook of Psychotherapy and Behavior Change,* 2nd ed. New York: Wiley, 1978.

MARMOR, J. Short-term dynamic psychotherapy. *American Journal of Psychiatry,* 1979, *136,* 149–155.

MASTERS, W. H., AND JOHNSON, V. *Human Sexual Response.* Boston: Little, Brown, 1966.

MASTERS, W. H., AND JOHNSON, V. *Human Sexual Inadequacy.* Boston: Little, Brown, 1970.

MEICHENBAUM, D. H. Cognitive factors in behavior modification: Modifying what clients say to themselves. In C. M. Franks and G. T. Wilson (Eds.), *Annual Review of Behavior Therapy: Theory and Practice.* New York: Brunner/Mazel, 1973.

MEICHENBAUM, D. H. *Cognitive Behavior Modification.* Morristown, NJ: General Learning Press, 1974.

MEICHENBAUM, D. H. Self instructional methods. In F. H. Kanfer and A. P. Goldstein (Eds.), *Helping People Change*. New York: Pergamon, 1975.

MEICHENBAUM, D. H. Teaching children self-control. In B. B. Lahey and A. E. Kazdin (Eds.), *Advances in Clinical Child Psychology*. New York: Plenum, 1979.

MELTZOFF, J., AND KORNREICH, M. *Research in Psychotherapy*. New York: Atherton Press, 1970.

MEYER, C. H. *Social Work Practice: A Response to the Urban Crisis*. New York: Free Press, 1970.

MINUCHIN, S. *Families and Family Therapy*. Cambridge, MA: Harvard University Press, 1974.

MINUCHIN, S., MONTALVO, B., GUERNEY, B., ROSMAN, B., AND SCHUMER, F. *Families of the Slums*. New York: Basic Books, 1967.

MINUCHIN, S., ROSMAN, B., AND BAKER, L. *Psychosomatic Families: Anorexia Nervosa in Context*. Cambridge MA: Harvard University Press, 1978.

MORENO, J. L. *Psychodrama*. New York: Beacon House, 1959.

MURRAY, E. J., AND JACOBSON, L. I. The nature of learning in traditional and behavioral psychotherapy. In A. E. Bergin and S. L. Garfield (Eds.), *Handbook of Psychotherapy and Behavior Change*, 1st Ed. New York: Wiley, 1971.

OLSEN, D. H. L. *Treating Relationships*. Lake Mills IA: Graphic Press, 1976.

PARAD, H. J. (Ed.) *Crisis Intervention: Selected Readings*. New York: Family Service Association of America, 1965.

PARAD, H. J., AND PARAD, L. J. A study of crisis-oriented planned short-term treatment, Parts I and II). *Social Casework*, 1968, *49*, 346–355 and 418–426.

PARAD, L. J. Short-term treatment: An overview of historical trends, issues and potentials. *Smith College Studies in Social Work*, 1971, *41*, 119–146.

PARLOFF, M. B. Can psychotherapy research guide the policy maker? *American Psychologist*, 1979, *34*, 296–306.

PARLOFF, M. B., WASKOW, I. E., AND WOLFE, B. E. Research on therapist variables in relation to process and outcome. In S. L. Garfield and A. E. Bergin (Eds.), *Handbook of Psychotherapy and Behavior Change,* 2nd ed. New York: Wiley, 1978.

PRUGER, R. Bureaucratic functioning as a social work skill. In B. L. Bauer and R. Federico (Eds.), *Educating the Baccalaureate Social Worker,* Cambridge, MA: Ballinger, 1978.

RABKIN, R. *Strategic Psychotherapy: Brief and Symptomatic Treatment.* New York: Basic Books, 1977.

RAIMY, V. *Misunderstandings of the Self: Cognitive Psychotherapy and the Misconception Hypothesis.* San Francisco: Jossey-Bass, 1975.

RAPAPORT, D. *The Collected Papers,* M. Gill (Ed.) New York: Basic Books, 1967.

RAPOPORT, L. Crisis intervention as a mode of treatment. In R. W. Roberts and R. H. Nee (Eds.), *Theories of Social Casework.* Chicago: University of Chicago Press, 1970.

RATHJEN, D. P., RATHJEN, E. D., AND HINIKER, A. A cognitive analysis of social performance: Implications for assessment and treatment. In J. P. Foreyt and D. P. Rathjen (Eds.), *Cognitive Behavior Therapy: Research and Application.* New York: Plenum, 1978.

REID, W. J. A test of the task-centered approach. *Social Work,* 1975, *22,* 3-9.

REID, W. J. *The Task-centered System.* New York: Columbia University Press, 1978.

REID, W. J., AND EPSTEIN, L. *Task-centered Casework.* New York: Columbia University Press, 1972.

REID, W. J., AND SHYNE, A. W. *Brief and Extended Casework.* New York: Columbia University Press, 1969.

RIPPLE, L., ALEXANDER, E., AND POLEMIS, B. *Motivation, Capacity and Opportunity.* Chicago: University of Chicago Press, 1964.

ROSE, S. *Group Therapy: A Behavioral Approach.* Englewood Cliffs, N.J.: Prentice-Hall, 1977.

RYAN, W. *Distress in the City.* Cleveland: Case Western Reserve University Press, 1969.

SALTER, A. *Conditioned Reflex Therapy.* New York: Creative Age, 1949.

SATIR, V. *Conjoint Family Therapy.* Palo Alto, CA: Science and Behavior Books, 1964.

SCHULMAN, L. *The Skills of Helping.* Itasca, IL: Peacock, 1979.

SHAPIRO, A. K., AND MORRIS, L. A. Placebo effects in medical and psychological therapies. In S. L. Garfield and A. E. Bergin (Eds.) *Handbook of Psychotherapy and Behavior Change,* 2nd ed. New York: Wiley, 1972.

SHAPIRO, D. *Neurotic Styles.* New York: Basic Books, 1965.

SHELTON, J. L. Murder strikes and panic follows: Can behavioral modification help? *Behavior Therapy,* 1973, *4,* 706–708.

SHELTON, J. L. The elimination of persistent stuttering by the use of homework assignments involving speech shadowing. *Behavior Therapy,* 1975, *6,* 392–393.

SHELTON, J. L. Instigation therapy: Using therapeutic homework to promote treatment gains. In A. P. Goldstein and F. H. Kanfer (Eds.), *Maximizing Treatment Gains: Transfer Enhancement in Psychotherapy.* New York: Academic Press, 1979.

SHELTON, J. L., AND ACKERMAN, J. M. *Homework in Counseling and Psychotherapy.* Springfield, IL: Thomas, 1974.

SIFNEOS, P. *Short-Term Psychotherapy and Emotional Crisis.* Cambridge, MA: Harvard University Press, 1972.

SLOANE, R. B., STAPLES, F. R., CRISTOL, A. H., YORKSTON, N. J., AND WHIPPLE, K. *Psychotherapy Versus Behavior Therapy.* Cambridge, MA: Harvard University Press, 1975.

SMITH, M. J. *When I Say No I Feel Guilty.* New York: Dial Press, 1975.

STAMPFL, T. G., AND LEVIS, D. J. Essentials of implosive therapy: A learning-theory-based psychodynamic behavior therapy. *Journal of Abnormal and Social Psychology,* 1967, *72,* 496–503.

STEIN, E. H., MURDAUGH, J., AND MacLEOD, J. A. Brief psychotherapy of psychiatric reactions to physical illness. In H. H. Barten (Ed.), *Brief Therapies.* New York: Behavioral Publications, 1971.

STEVENSON, I. Direct instigation of behavioral changes in psychotherapy. *Archives of General Psychiatry,* 1959, *61,* 99–117.

STEVENSON, I. Processes of "spontaneous" recovery from the psychoneuroses. *American Journal of Psychiatry,* 1961, *117,* 1057–1064.

STRONG, S. Social psychological factors in psychotherapy. In A. E.

Bergin and S. L. Garfield (Eds.), *Handbook of Psychotherapy and Behavior Change,* 1st ed. New York: Wiley, 1971.

STRUPP, H. H. Psychotherapy research and practice: An overview. In S. L. Garfield and A. E. Bergin (Eds.), *Handbook of Psychotherapy and Behavior Change,* 2nd ed. New York: Wiley, 1978.

STORROW, A. H. *Introduction to Scientific Psychiatry.* New York: Appleton, 1967.

SULLIVAN, H. S. *The Interpersonal Theory of Psychiatry.* New York: Norton, 1953.

SULLIVAN, H. S. *The Psychiatric Interview.* New York: Norton, 1954.

TRUAX, C. B., AND CARKHUFF, R. R. *Toward Effective Counseling and Psychotherapy.* Chicago: Aldine, 1967.

TRUAX, C. B., AND MITCHELL, K. M. Research on certain therapist interpersonal skills in relation to process and outcome. In A. E. Bergin and S. L. Garfield (Eds.), *Handbook of Psychotherapy and Behavior Change,* 1st ed. New York: Wiley, 1971.

TURNER, F. J. Some considerations on the place of theory in current social work practice. In F. J. Turner (Ed.), *Social Work Treatment: Interlocking Theoretical Approaches.* New York: Free Press, 1974.

TURNER, F. J. *Psychosocial Therapy.* New York: Free Press, 1978.

TURNER, F. J. (Ed.). *Social Work Treatment: Interlocking Theoretical Approaches,* 2nd ed. New York: Free Press, 1979.

VATTANO, A. Self-management procedures for coping with stress. *Social Work,* 1978, *23,* 113–120.

VERNY, T. R. Analysis of attrition rates in a psychiatric outpatient clinic. *Psychiatric Quarterly,* 1970, *44,* 37–48.

WACHTEL, PAUL L. *Psychoanalysis and Behavior Therapy: Toward an Integration.* New York: Basic Books, 1977.

WALEN, S. R., DiGUISEPPE, R., AND WESSLER, R. L. *A Practitioner's Guide to Rational-emotive Therapy.* New York: Oxford University Press, 1980.

WASSERMAN, S. Ego psychology. In F. J. Turner (Ed.) *Social Work Treatment: Interlocking Theoretical Approaches.* New York: Free Press, 1974.

WATSON, P. *War on the Mind: The Military Uses and Abuses of Psychology.* New York: Basic Books, 1978.

WATTIE, B. Evaluation of short-term casework in a family agency. *Social Casework*, 1973, *54*, 609–616.

WAXENBERG, B. Therapist's empathy, regard and genuineness as factors in staying in or dropping out of short-term, time-limited family therapy. *Dissertation Abstracts International*, 1973, *34*, 1288B.

WAXER, P. H. Short-term group psychotherapy: Some principles and techniques. *International Journal of Group Psychotherapy*, 1977, *27*, 33–42.

WEINBERGER, G. Brief therapy with children and their parents. In H. H. Barten (Ed.) *Brief Therapies*. New York: Behavioral Publications, 1971.

WEISMAN, A. Industrial social work: Linkage technology. *Social Casework*, 1976, *57*, 50–54.

WELLS, R. A. (Ed.). Short-term treatment: An annotated bibliography, 1945–1974. *Journal Supplement Abstract Service: Selected Catalogue of Documents in Psychology*, 1976, *6*, 13–14.

WELLS, R. A. Engagement techniques in family therapy. *International Journal of Family Therapy*, 1980, *2*, 75–94.

WELLS, R. A. The empirical base of family therapy: Practice implications. In E. R. Tolson and W. J. Reid (Eds.), *Models of Family Treatment*. New York: Columbia University Press, in press.

WELLS, R. A., AND DEZEN, A. E. The results of family therapy revisited: The nonbehavioral methods. *Family Process*, 1978, *17*, 251–274.

WELLS, R. A., AND FIGUREL, J. A. Techniques of structured communication training. *The Family Coordinator*, 1979, *28*, 273–281.

WELLS, R. A., FIGUREL, J. A., AND McNAMEE, P. Communication training vs. conjoint marital therapy. *Social Work Research and Abstracts*, 1977, *13*, 31–39.

WHITE, R. *Ego and Reality in Psychoanalytic Theory*. New York: International Universities Press, 1963.

WITTMAN, M. Preventitive social work: A goal for practice and intervention. *Social Work*, 1961, *6*, 19–27.

WOLPE, J. Foreword. In C. M. Franks (Ed.), *Behavior Therapy: Appraisal and Status*. New York: McGraw-Hill, 1969.

WOLPE, J. *The Practice of Behavior Therapy*, 2nd ed. New York: Pergamon, 1973.

WOLPE, J., AND LAZARUS, A. A. *Behavior Therapy Techniques.* New York: Pergamon, 1966.

WOOD, K. Casework effectiveness: A new look at the research evidence. *Social Work,* 1978, *23,* 437–459.

ZUK, G. Values and family therapy. *Psychotherapy: Theory, Research, and Practice,* 1978, *15,* 48–55.

Index

Index